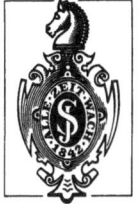

Robert Sigal
D. Doyon · Ph. Halimi · H. Atlan

Magnetic Resonance Imaging

Basis for Interpretation

Translated by
S. Assénat and R. Sigal

With 122 Illustrations

Springer-Verlag
Berlin Heidelberg New York
London Paris Tokyo

R. Sigal, M. D. · D. Doyon, M. D. · Ph. Halimi, M. D.
Service de Radiologie
78 rue du général Leclerc
F-94270 Le Kremlin Bicêtre, France

H. Atlan, M. D., Ph. D
Department of Medical Biophysics
Hadassah University Hospital
Jerusalem, Israel

ISBN-13 : 978-3-642-73039-9   e-ISBN-13 : 978-3-642-73037-5
DOI: 10.1007/978-3-642-73037-5

Library of Congress Cataloging-in-Publication Data.
Sigal, Robert, 1956-   . Magnetic resonance imaging : basis for interpretation / Robert Sigal.
    p.   cm. Bibliography: p.   1. Magnetic resonance imaging. I. Title.
    RC78.7.N83S55   1988   616. 07'57 – dc19   87-28541

© Springer-Verlag Berlin Heidelberg 1988
Softcover reprint of the hardcover 1st edition 1988

Reproduction of the figures: Gustav Dreher GmbH, Stuttgart

2127/3130-543210

Foreword

Magnetic Resonance Imaging (MRI) is a rapidly evolving technique which is having a significant impact on medical imaging. Only a few years ago, although Nuclear Magnetic Resonance (NMR) was well known as an important analytical technique in the field of chemical analysis, it was effectively unknown in medical circles.

Following the initial work of PAUL LAUTERBUR and RAYMOND DAMADIAN in the early 1970s demonstrating that it was possible to use NMR to produce images, progress in the medical fields was relatively slow. Recently, however, with the availability of commercial systems, progress has been very rapid, with increasing acceptance of MRI as a basic imaging technique, and the development of exciting new applications.

MRI is a relatively complex technique. First, the image depends on many more intrinsic and extrinsic parameters than it does of in techniques like X-radiography and computed tomography, and secondly, the intrinsic parameters such as T1 and T2 are conceptually complex, involving ideas not usually described in traditional medical imaging courses. In order to produce good MR images efficiently, and to obtain the maximum information from them, it is necessary to appreciate, if not to fully understand, these parameters. Furthermore, knowledge of how the image is produced helps in appreciating the origin of the artifacts sometimes found in MRI due to effects like patient motion and fluid flow.

Dr. SIGAL has used his experience, gained as one of the first European Radiologists to become intensively involved with MRI in a clinical setting, to produce a clear basic guide to MRI. The book leads the reader, in a simple tutorial style, through the basic physics of MRI and develops criteria for choosing, for example, the correct pulse sequence for a specific study. The significance of these, criteria is illustrated by many examples drawn from the authors experience. This book will provide a valuable introduction to the subject, both for those who plan to use the technique extensively in the future and for those who simply feel that they should understand the basics of this new imaging modality.

December 1987   DEREK SHAW, BSc. PhD.

Preface

This book is an introduction to Magnetic Resonance Imaging (MRI) for radiologists and doctors wishing to understand for themselves the results of examinations as well as the ever greater amount of literature published on this new technique. It aims at helping anyone unfamiliar with MRI to begin to interpret the images. Therefore, I only mention the basic principles that should be known for this interpretation. Since my objective was mainly didactic, I sometimes had to use educational patterns, some of which are only an approximation of physical reality.

I intentionally pass over the technological aspect of imaging itself as far as it has no direct effect on interpretation (however, I briefly mention signal localization in an appendix), as well as techniques, such as spectroscopy and non-hydrogen imaging, which are not yet part of "routine" MRI.

Eight exercises, allowing the readers to test the knowledge they have acquired, are presented at the end of this book.

Acknowledgements. Almost all of the MRI images in this book were made using the high-field MRI system (SIGNA, General Electric) of the Centre Inter Etablissements de Résonance Magnétique (CIERM) in Bicêtre Hospital, Paris. I am grateful to the chairman of the CIERM, Professor A. DESGREZ, for receiving me and helping me complete this work. This book could never have been written without the efficiency and helpfulness of the CIERM technologists. I thank D. VANEL, P. LASJAUNIAS, A. LEROY-WILLIG, A. ROCHE, S. TRAN DINH, I. IDY, J. BENMAÏR (Elscint Company) and R. BROSSEL (Schering Laboratories) for the images they generously lent to me. D. LACLEF and J. M. MEIGNÉ ensured photographic processing with great talent. Mrs. C. VACHON was a precious help in drawing some of the figures. Professor V. BISMUTH accepted the task of reviewing the manuscript; I thank him warmly for this. My friends C. BLAS, G. POYLECOT and J. E. LEFÈVRE also gave me helpful advice. I thank D. SHAW and B. WILLINSKY for assistance with the translation. Lastly, I wish to express my gratitude to J. BITTOUN, with whom I discussed the scientific aspects of this book.

December 1987   ROBERT SIGAL, M. D.

Table of Contents

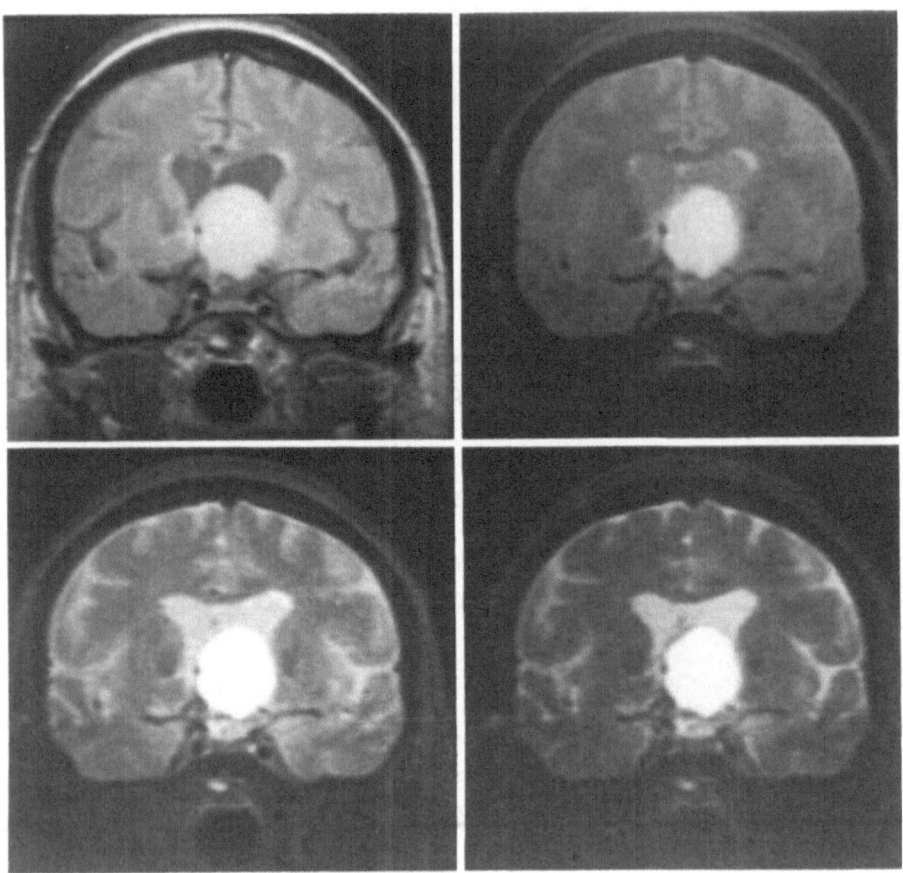

Fig. 1.1. Coronal sections of the brain. Suprasellar craniopharyngioma

Chapter 1 **Introduction**

Even more than any other imaging technique, nuclear magnetic resonance (NMR) requires an understanding of the basic principles in order to be able to interpret the images correctly (Fig. 1.1).

Routine clinical NMR imaging is based on the study of the hydrogen nucleus. This nucleus consists of one particle: the *proton* (Fig. 1.2).

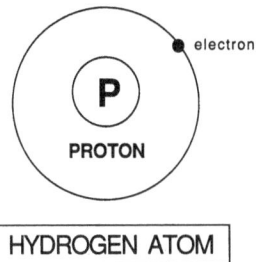

Fig. 1.2

HYDROGEN ATOM

To simplify, it is assumed that "protons" implicitly means "hydrogen nuclei" (although the nuclei of all other atoms also have protons).

What makes hydrogen nuclei the objects of choice for NMR imaging is, among other factors, their great abundance in the human body, especially in the form of water molecules.

This concern with nuclei lies behind the use of the term *"nuclear* magnetic resonance". Since the word "nuclear" can lead to confusion with radioactive phenomena, the term "magnetic resonance imaging" (MRI) is preferred.

The basic principle of MRI may be represented as follows:

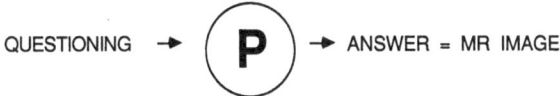

QUESTIONING → (P) → ANSWER = MR IMAGE

Fig. 1.3

MRI consists in questioning the protons.
The protons answer by generating the MR image.

Questioning the protons occurs by exciting them with a given amount of *energy*. This energy is carried by electromagnetic waves (Fig. 1.4).

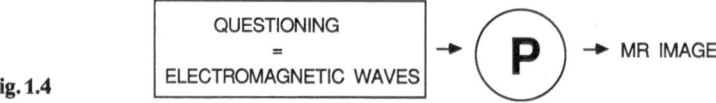

Fig. 1.4

The wavelengths used in MRI are similar to those used in radiocommunication (hence the term "radiofrequency waves"). Therefore, they represent very low-energy radiation (Fig. 1.5).

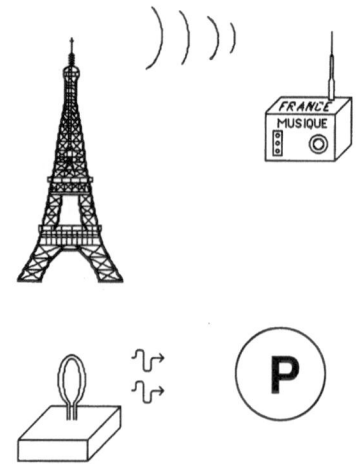

Fig. 1.5

In fact, there are several ways of questioning protons. Each kind of questioning generates a different image for the *same slice* (Fig. 1.6).

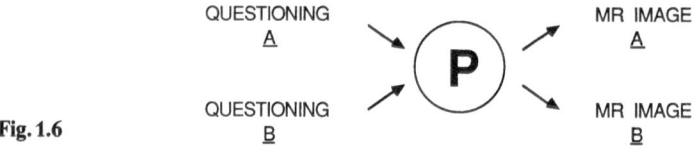

Fig. 1.6

Figure 1.7 shows three sagittal sections of the *same patient* made during the *same session* of imaging. According to the type of questioning, the appearance of the different kinds of tissue changes: on the first image, for example, the cerebrospinal fluid appears dark grey, whereas it is light grey on the second image and white on the third one. On the contrary, a colloid cyst of the third ventricle (▶) is white on the first image, and black on the third one.

Fig. 1.8 shows another example: these three axial sections were performed across the upper part of the abdomen in the same patient. There is a space-occupying lesion in the liver (▶). According to the way of questioning the protons, it looks black, white, or cannot be distinguished from the adjacent parenchyma.

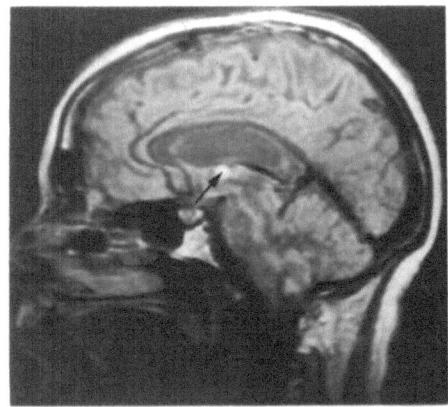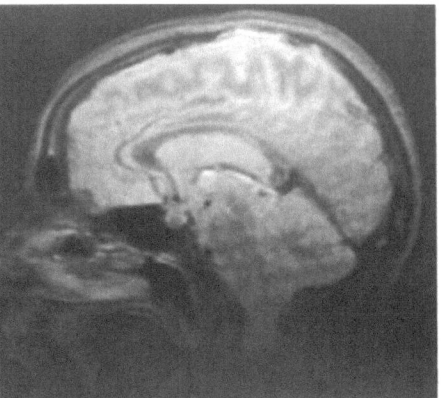

Fig. 1.7

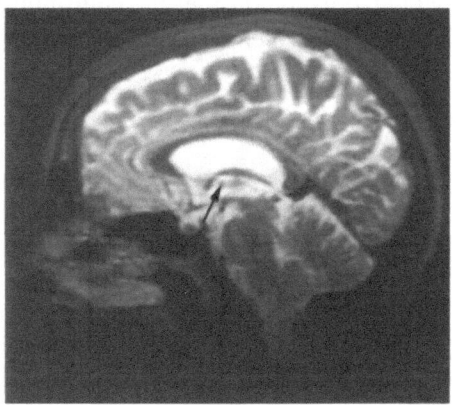

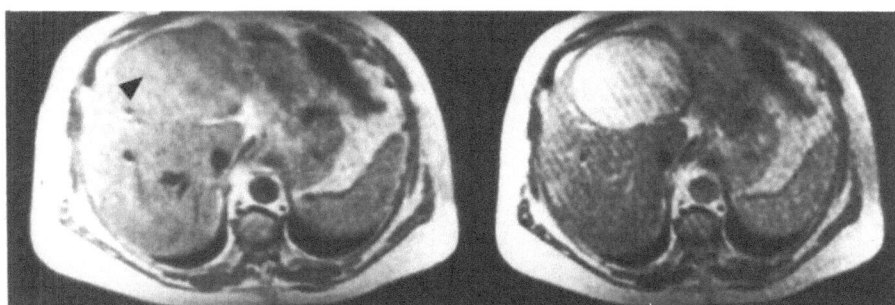

Fig. 1.8

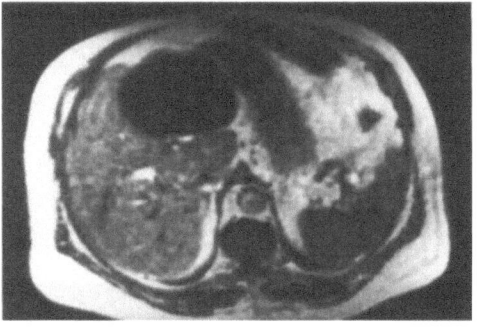

3

Protons may be compared with a dancer; in both cases, the behavior observed depends on two factors, which can be termed "intrinsic" and "extrinsic":

For the dancer – personal qualities
                – music
For the protons – tissue parameters
                – acquisition parameters

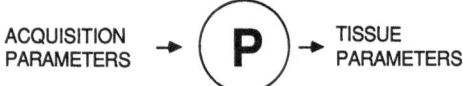

Fig. 1.9

These tissue and acquisition parameters will be the object of our study in the Chaps. 2 and 3. This will lead us to consider the contribution of MRI to diagnosis (Chap. 4) and the way in which an MRI examination should be performed (Chap. 5).

Chapter 2   Tissue Parameters

Let us return to the basic principle of MRI (Fig. 2.1):

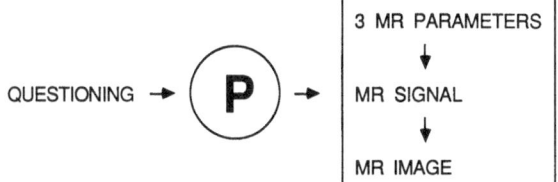

QUESTIONING → (**P**) → 3 MR PARAMETERS
↓
MR SIGNAL
↓
MR IMAGE

Fig. 2.1

Once excited, the protons induce signals.
The MR image is made of a set of signals.
The signal depends on *three* main parameters.

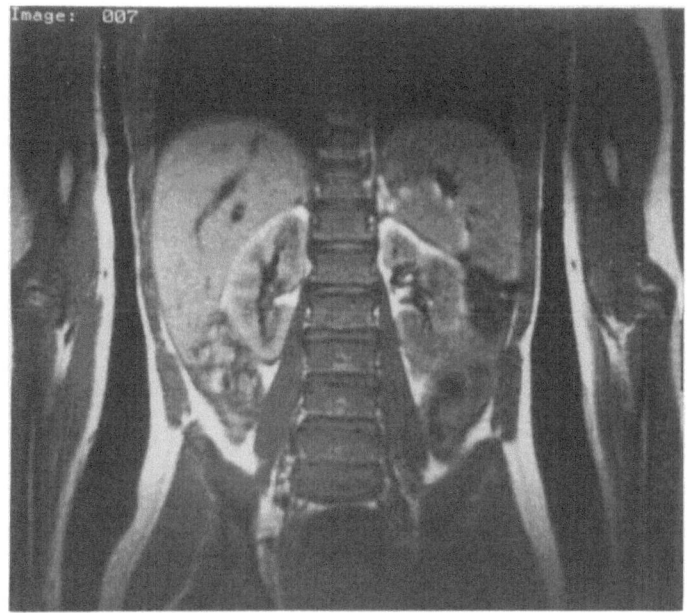

Fig. 2.2. Coronal section across the abdomen and the upper limbs

In conventional radiology or computerized tomography, the signal (and therefore the image) depends on one parameter only: the X-ray beam attenuation coefficient. In MRI, however, the image is generated by three factors. Therefore:

Understanding the formation of MR images (and thus being able to interpret them) involves being able to juggle with all three parameters.

MRI is a complex tool for diagnosis, but is potentially very efficient.

The three parameters are:

ρ **PROTON DENSITY**

T1
)   **RELAXATION TIMES**

Fig. 2.3   T2

Proton density, represented by the Greek letter ρ (rho), describes the number of protons in one volume unit. Proton density is very low in air, where there are few protons that can be excited: for that reason, there is no MR signal (Fig. 2.4).

The density of protons hardly varies according to the kind of soft tissue; in other words, ρ plays little part in generating contrast. As a matter of fact, ρ is a sort of foundation on which the determining elements of MRI, i.e., the relaxation times, are built. When it decreases (or drops to zero), no relaxation time can be found because there are no protons to be excited: this is the case with air.

Relaxation times are the fundamental parameters of MRI: let us try to explain them simply.

Protons may be considered as tiny bar magnets and thus as having a North pole and a South pole (Fig. 2.5).

NORTH

Fig. 2.5   SOUTH

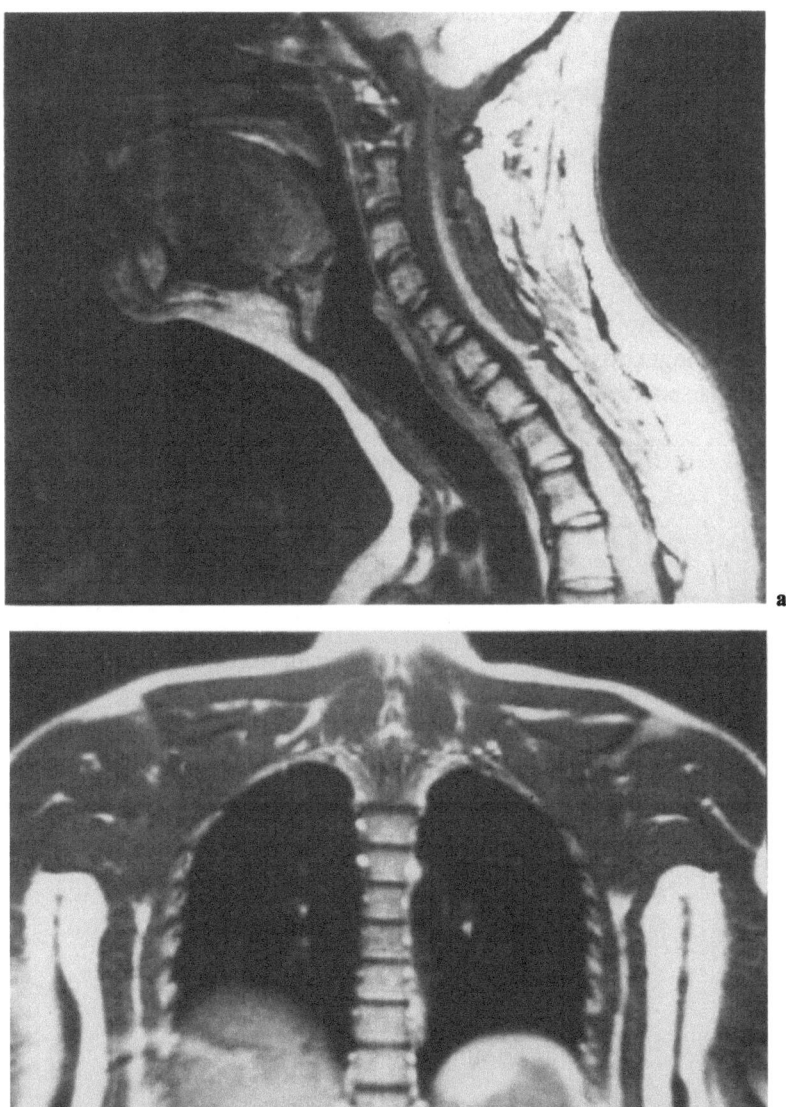

Fig. 2.4. a Midsagittal section of the cervical area (postoperative aspect of the cord). **b** Coronal
section of the thorax behind the heart. The trachea and the lungs appear black.

In the absence of a magnetic field, the protons are oriented at random in the organism (Fig. 2.6).

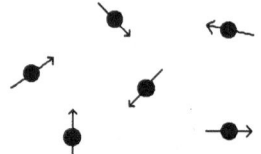

Fig. 2.6

When subjected to an intense magnetic field, the protons orient in the direction of this magnetic field and reach a state of equilibrium (Fig. 2.7). The magnetic field is represented by Bo.[1]

EQUILIBRIUM

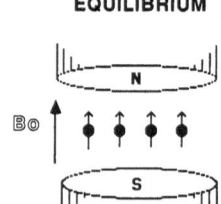

Fig. 2.7

Transmission of energy to the protons forces them to flip from their equilibrium position. (This energy is carried by electromagnetic waves (see Fig. 1.4) and delivered by a transmitter coil). The protons are then said to be excited (Fig. 2.8).[2]

EXCITATION

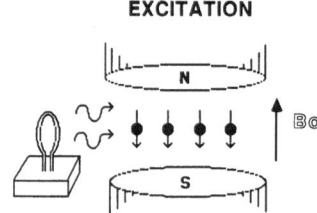

Fig. 2.8

When excitation is interrupted, the protons spontaneously return to their equilibrium position: they relax. During relaxation, the protons induce MR signals generating the MR image (Fig. 2.9).[3] *Therefore relaxation is the return of protons to equilibrium after excitation.*

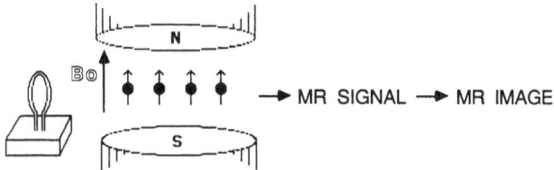

Fig. 2.9

In fact, overall relaxation can be described in terms of two events:

T1: spin-lattice relaxation time,
T2: spin-spin relaxation time.

In order to describe T1 and T2, the M (magnetization) vector has to be used.

As we have seen, protons behave like tiny magnets. Therefore, a magnetization vector can be attributed to them, as to any other magnet. The intensity of each vector has a microscopic value, which cannot be measured. However, the intensity of a collection of vectors can be measured: this is macroscopic magnetization (M vector) (Fig. 2.10 a).

---

[1] Magnetic field intensity is indicated in Tesla (T; SI unit) or Gauss (G; 1 T = 10000 G).
The magnetic fields of the currently available MRI systems range from 0.02 to 2 T, whereas Earth's magnetic field is lower than 1 G.

There are three types of magnets:

Permanent magnets: though simple and cheap to run, they are still extremely heavy and do not generate high fields.

Resistive magnets: these are electromagnets, the magnetic field being generated by an electric current flowing through a coil. They have two major drawbacks: high electric and water consumption (cooling) and generated fields that are difficult to raise above 0.15 T.

Superconductive magnets: these are also electromagnets, made of materials with no electric resistance when placed at a temperature close to absolute zero (−273 °C). They consume no power and allow stable and very high fields to be generated. Their major drawback is running costs (cryogens); however, they are more and more commonly used.

[2] The protons are also said to be in "antiparallel" position. In quantum physics, there are only two positions likely to be occupied by protons subjected to a magnetic field: parallel (lower energy level) or antiparallel (upper energy level). Although the difference between the two populations is very small, we will, nevertheless, focus on it. At equilibrium, there is a small excess of protons in the parallel position; excitation may equalize the two populations, or generate a small excess in the antiparallel position. On the other hand, the difference between the two energy levels is constant (and dependent on the intensity of Bo). When the transmitted energy exactly matches this difference, the energy transferred to the protons reaches its maximal value: *resonance* occurs between the exciting system and the excited protons.

[3] These signals are also electromagnetic waves that are collected by a receiver coil. The same coil is often used for transmission and reception.

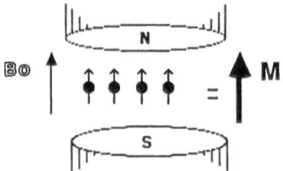

Fig. 2.10a

The M vector therefore represents the resultant of the protons taken into account, the orientation of which, according to Bo, depends on the proportion of protons in the parallel and antiparallel position (see note 2, p. 9) (Fig. 2.10b, c).

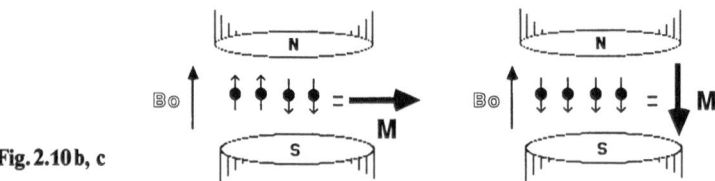

Fig. 2.10b, c

Equilibrium: The M vector is in line with the magnetic field Bo. The direction of Bo defines the longitudinal axis (Fig. 2.11a).

Excitation: The energy supply creates excitation leading to a flip of M (90° here). M is then perpendicular to its equilibrium position: it lies in a transverse plane (Fig. 2.11b).

Relaxation: Relaxation occurs when excitation ceases. It is made up of two phenomena, T1 and T2 (Fig. 2.11c).

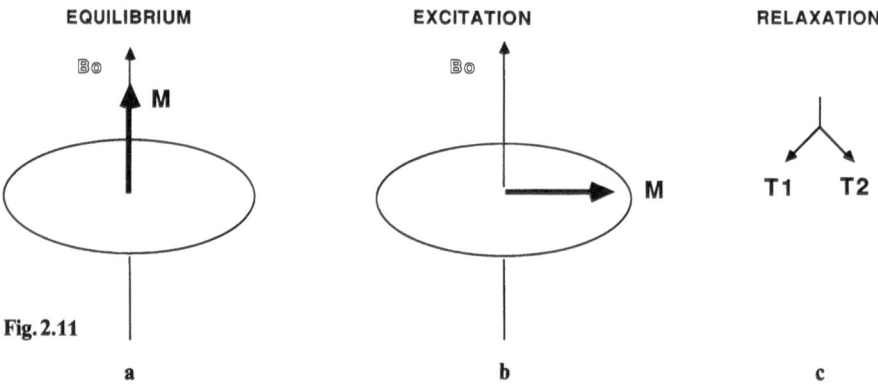

Fig. 2.11

T1 *(spin-lattice relaxation time)*

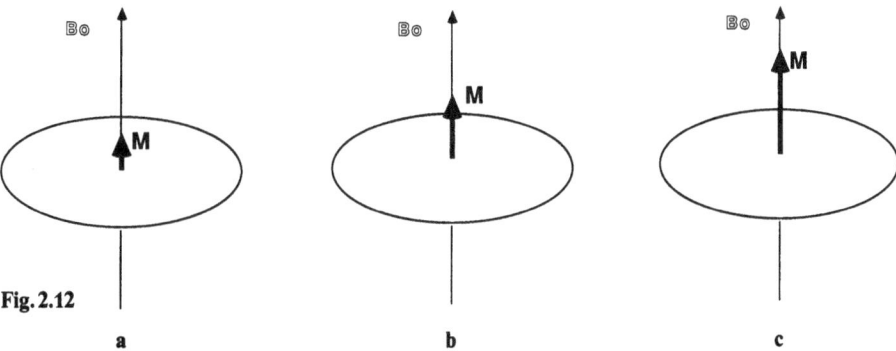

Fig. 2.12

a   b   c

T1 characterizes the return of the M vector to equilibrium along the longitudinal axis defined by Bo (Fig 2.12) (and is also called "longitudinal relaxation time" for that reason).

In order to understand the meaning of T1, let us examine the terminology:

Spin: term from quantum physics, referring to the fact that protons spin at high speed.

Lattice: term used in solid state physics and chemistry. By extension, in MRI, it means the set of atoms surrounding an excited proton. It is therefore the molecular environment of a proton, and in a wider sense its biological environment (water, fat, etc.).

Thus T1, or spin-lattice relaxation time, is the result of interaction between *protons* (acting through their spinning properties) and the whole *environment*.

More precisely, T1 is characteristic for the efficiency of the environment for absorbing the energy of excited protons during relaxation: short when the environment has a high efficiency for absorbing energy as in the case of fat; long in the opposite case, as in pure water.

The return to equilibrium of two different kinds of tissue can be plotted as a function of time (Fig. 2.13).

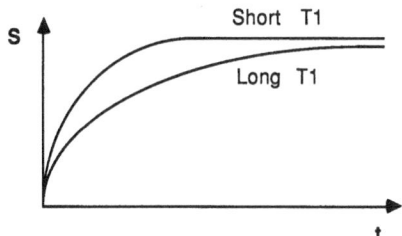

Fig. 2.13

Note that:

This return corresponds to an exponential increase.

Initially, i.e., during relaxation, both curves are clearly separated: T1 contrast is therefore enhanced.

After a certain time, when relaxation has occurred, both curves plateau at the same maximum. At this time, the signal depends on the density of protons, which is practically equal in both kinds of tissue: the contrast observed at this point is therefore low.

T2 *(spin-spin relaxation time).*

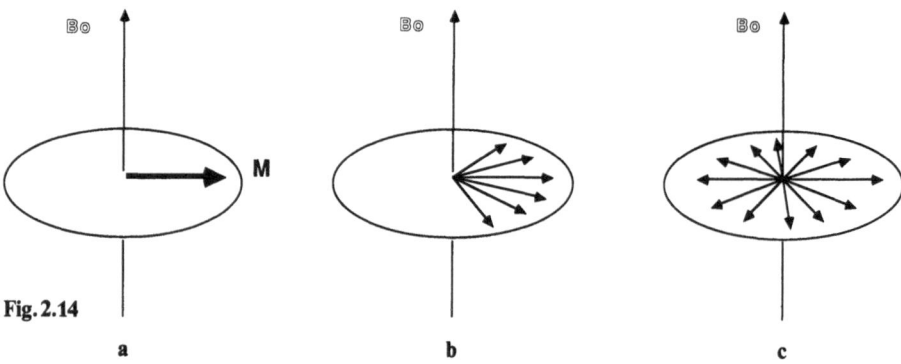

Fig. 2.14

a   b   c

T2 characterizes the disappearance of the M vector in the transverse plane perpendicular to Bo (Fig. 2.14) (for that reason, T2 is also called "transverse relaxation time"):

(a) Immediately after the delivery of energy, the M vector is perpendicular to Bo, as we have just seen. Moreover, the protons also have the same direction: they are said to be "in phase."

(b) The protons, exerting microvariations on each other's magnetic fields, get dephased: there is a loss of phase coherence.

(c) After a given time, dephasing is complete: the resultant of all the vectors is zero in the transverse (i.e. perpendicular to Bo) plane. The signal has vanished.

12

Thus, T2 is called spin-spin relaxation time because it is the *result of interactions between neighboring protons.*

More precisely, since each proton is a tiny magnet, it creates a micromagnetic field more or less disturbing the neighboring protons, thus leading to a loss of phase coherence. The tissues in which there are relatively significant microvariations added to Bo rapidly lose phase coherence: T2 is short. This is the case with fat. The microvariations have relatively little effect in other tissues: T2 is long, as for instance in pure water.

The loss of signal corresponding to the effect of T2 can be plotted for two different tissues (Fig. 2.15).

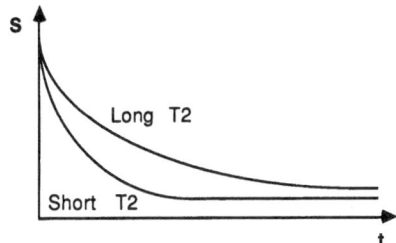

Fig. 2.15

Note that:

Decrease is exponential.

The two curves are practically superimposed at the beginning, since microvariations have as yet had no effect.

The relative effects of microvariations in each tissue appear after a short time: the two curves part and the T2 contrast then observed between both tissues is high.

After a certain time, dephasing is complete for both substances, and there is no more signal.

Note 1: We have just seen that two effects are obtained when protons are excited: (1) the M vector flips from its equilibrium position, and (2) the protons get in phase. The second effect indicates that the protons are not in phase when they are at equilibrium. The process can be represented as follows:

Protons spin on themselves. But they also rotate around the axis of Bo (in a so-called "precession" movement). However, the axis of this movement is not parallel to Bo but at a certain angle to it. Moreover, protons at equilibrium are not in phase but have different directions. They are evenly distributed in a cone ("precession cone"), the axis of which is Bo. The M vector is the result of this balanced distribution of protons (Fig. 2.16).

13

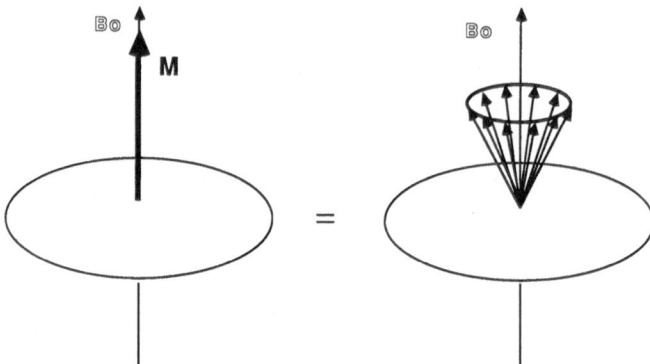

Fig. 2.16

When receiving energy, protons regroup in one direction of the precession cone: they get in phase. Simultaneously, the M vector flips, as the proportion between protons in the parallel and antiparallel position changes (Fig. 2.17).

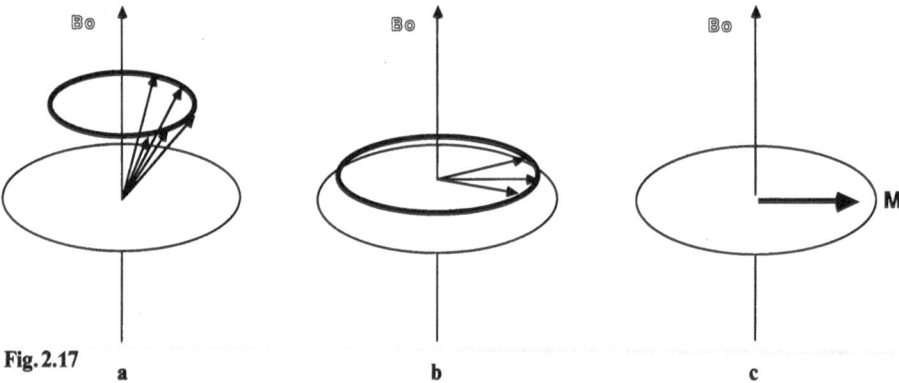

Fig. 2.17   a   b   c

During relaxation, there is a progressive return to equilibrium. This means that the protons progressively return to their uniform position around Bo: the loss of phase coherence has actually occurred (some protons precess faster than others). Simultaneously, M returns to its equilibrium position (Fig. 2.18).

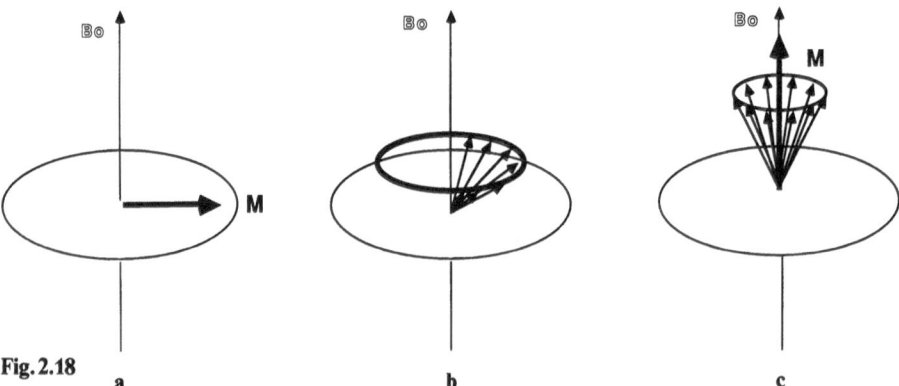

Fig. 2.18   a   b   c

Note 2: If the field Bo is not uniform, the protons also get out of phase with one another. This is not a natural process, it is an instrumental artifact. Thus, transverse magnetization is lost by two processes: external T2 effects (Bo inhomogeneities) and internal or intrinsic T2 effects (true spin-spin relaxation) (see consequences p. 25)

14

Thus relaxation times depend on the *biological state* of tissues, and in just the same way that different people vary in weight and height, *tissues have different T1 and T2.*

Table 2.1

	T1 (ms)	T2 (ms)
Normal myocardium	690	40
Irreversible myocardial injury (Bo = 0.35 Tesla)	764	46

From: McNamara MT et al. (1986) Differentiation of reversible and irreversible myocardial injury by MR imaging with and without gadolinium-DTPA. Radiology 158: 765–769

The normal myocardium and the acutely injured myocardium have different tissue, i.e., molecular, composition: they have neither the same T1 nor the same T2.

T1 and T2 are constant in a given tissue in a given state. The ranges of T1 and T2 in biological tissue are as follows (in milliseconds):

T1: 300–2000 ms
T2: 30–150 ms

Let us now return to MR images. Figure 2.19 shows an axial section of the brain at the level of the ventricles.

The intensity of each point in the image is the result of a "blend" of the parameters ρ, T1 and T2; however, it is possible to monitor the proportions of ρ, T1 and T2.

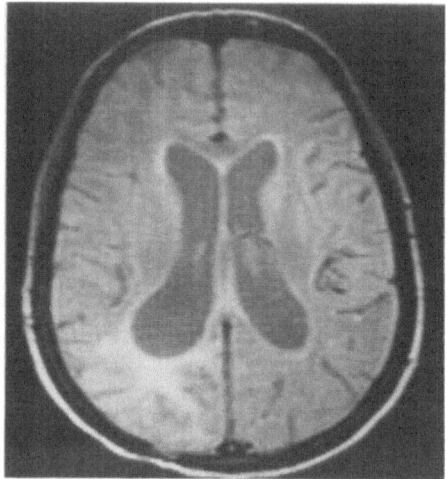

Fig. 2.19

Figure 2.20 provides an illustration of this: in the same patient and in the same plane, T1 contrast (Fig. 2.20a), then T2 contrast (Fig. 2.20b) have been enhanced.

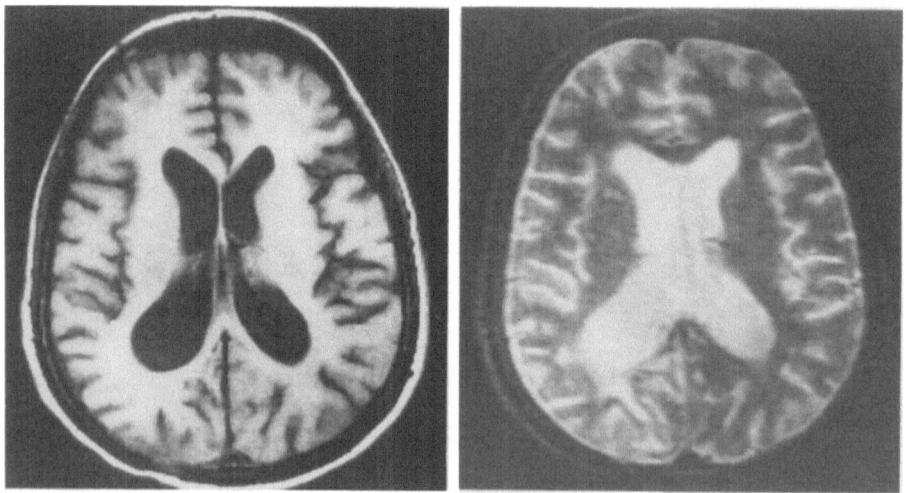

Fig. 2.20 a, b

The three parameters may be compared with the members of a music trio: usually, the three players play together, producing an ensemble. If two of them play softly, however, the melody of the remaining musician can be better heard.

We are the director of the trio: we can ask one or another musician to play pianissimo or fortissimo. The doctor performing the MRI examination also decides which of ρ, T1 and T2 will be the dominating factor. Our "scores" are called *pulse sequences*.

Chapter 3   Acquisition Parameters (Pulse Sequences)

What Is a Pulse?

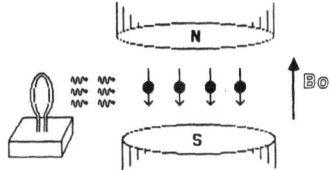

We have seen that protons are excited by a given amount of energy supplied in the form of low-energy electromagnetic waves or "radiofrequency waves" (see p. 2). This energy is not emitted by the transmitter coil continuously, but in short *pulses*. For that reason, we say that protons are excited by radiofrequency wave pulses, or, for short, RF pulses.

We know that the protons can be represented by the magnetization vector **M.**

With no RF pulse: Fig. 3.2a   Bo↑   ↑ **M**

the **M** vector is in equilibrium and parallel to the magnetic field Bo.

Two main RF pulses are used:

(1) 90° pulse

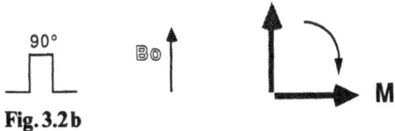

Fig. 3.2b

M rotates to an angle of 90° to its equilibrium position.

19

(2) 180° pulse

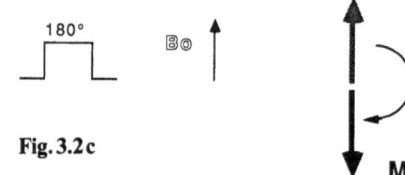

Fig. 3.2 c

this can be the initial pulse (*inversion* of **M** with relation to Bo)

or a pulse following a 90° pulse.

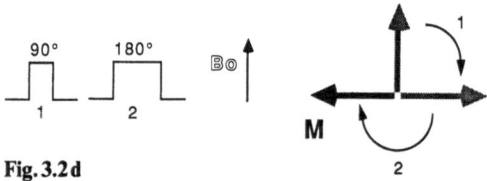

Fig. 3.2 d

What Is a Pulse Sequence?

A pulse sequence is a succession of RF pulses at varying time intervals.

Fig. 3.3 a

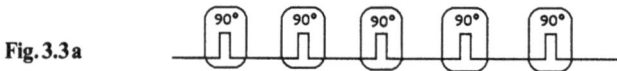

Here is a sequence that is repeated 5 times. Each sequence is made of one 90° pulse only. (By convention, we box each sequence, whatever the number of pulses.)

Fig. 3.3 b

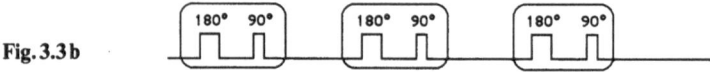

Here, the sequence is repeated 3 times. Each sequence consists of two pulses: 180° then 90°.

Fig. 3.3 c

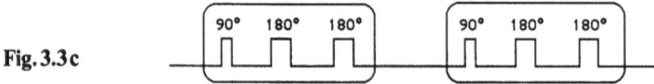

Lastly, here is a three-pulse sequence, 90° – 180° – 180°, repeated twice.

Time Intervals

Three time intervals should be defined: the first between sequences, the other two within a sequence.

Repetition time (TR) (Fig. 3.4a). This is the time interval between the beginning of a sequence and the beginning of the following one. *The duration of TR is chosen by the operator.*

Fig. 3.4a

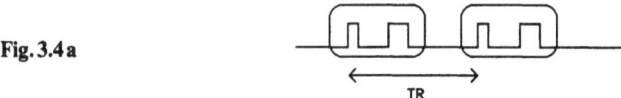

Inversion time (TI) and echo time (TE) (Fig. 3.4b). The meaning of these intervals will be explained below (p. 23 and 30). *Their durations are also determined by the operator.*

Fig. 3.4b

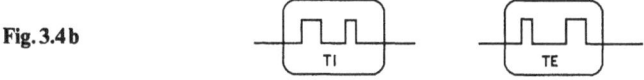

Sequences Used in MRI

Essentially, three pulse sequences can be described:

Partial saturation (PS)
Spin echo (SE)
Inversion recovery (IR)

We will consider (a) the structure (RF pulses and time intervals), and (b) the practical use (tissue parameters made visible) of each sequence. We will see that the contribution of the three sequences to diagnosis is not the same: the sequence most used nowadays is the spin echo.

Fast imaging sequences have appeared recently and are becoming more and more important, for, as their name suggest, they make it possible to shorten scanning time. We will close this chapter with a description of this new type of sequences.

Partial Saturation

Structure

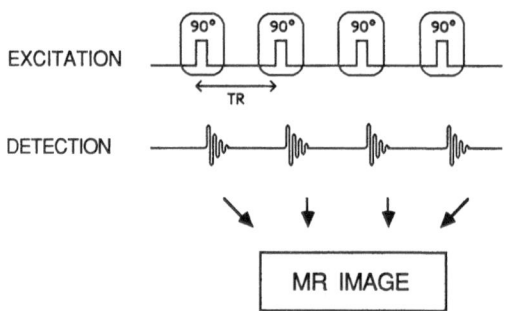

Fig. 3.5

Excitation: Each pulse sequence includes one 90° RF pulse only.
The only time interval described is therefore TR.

Detection: The protons induce a signal after each RF pulse.
The addition of all the signals received yields the MR image (see Fig. 2.1).

Use

Partial saturation allows visualization of two MR parameters, ρ and T1. Monitoring TR makes it possible to control the respective proportion of ρ and T1 effects:

When TR is very long (a few seconds), image contrast is essentially generated by ρ: the image obtained is said to be "ρ-weighted".

When TR is shorter, the effect of T1 on the image is greater.

In practice TR $\geqslant$ 2500 ms is rarely used practically, because (a) the examination time increases in proportion to TR (see p. 64), and (b) ρ varies much less than T1 according to the kind of soft tissue: T1-weighted images therefore allow for better contrast than ρ-weighted ones.

To summarize:[1]

$$TR \geqslant 2000 \text{ ms} \leftrightarrow \rho \text{ image}$$
$$100 \text{ ms} \leqslant TR \leqslant 1500 \text{ ms} \leftrightarrow T1 \text{ image}$$

Spin Echo

Spin echo is the most frequently used pulse sequence.

Structure

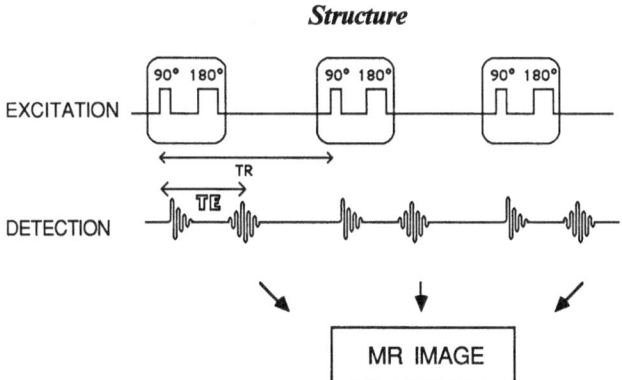

Fig. 3.6

Excitation: Each pulse sequence is composed of two RF pulses: 90° then 180°. Two time intervals can be described:

TR: repetition time
TE: echo time

Detection: In order to explain the meaning of TE, let us analyze the sequence:

The first RF pulse (90°) produces a signal which is not directly used by the machine to generate an image.

---

[1] The influence of TR is easy to understand if one considers the curves previously shown in Fig. 2.13.

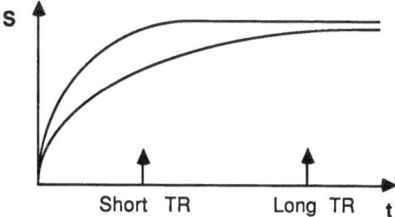

Fig. 3.7

When a given sequence is performed, relaxation is "photographed" at a given time, this moment being defined by TR:

If a short TR is chosen, the image is taken at a moment when T1 contrast between different kinds of tissue is enhanced.
If TR is long, the "photograph" shows tissue having returned to equilibrium; the image obtained is then ρ-weighted and the contrast between the different kinds of tissue is low.
But when TR becomes extremely short, the signal is weak, leading to poor-quality images. For this reason, TR shorter than 200 ms is rarely used.

23

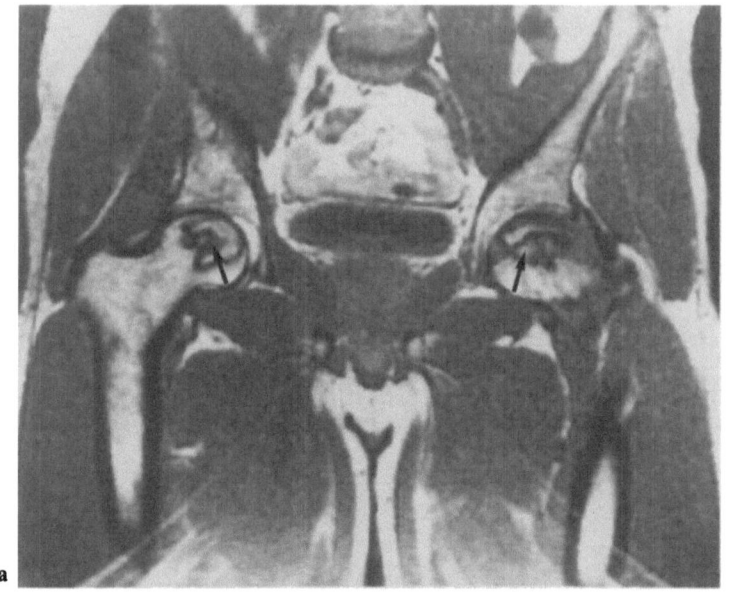

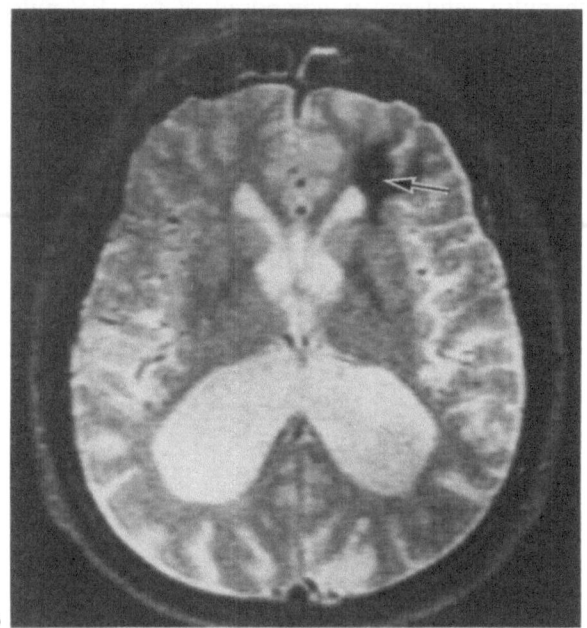

Fig. 3.8. a Frontal section at the level of the femoral heads (→) and the hip joints. Bilateral osteonecrosis of the femoral heads. TR = 500 ms, TE = 20 ms (T1 weighting). **b** Axial section of the brain. Ventricular enlargement, cortical atrophy, chronic left frontal haematoma (↔). TR = 2500 ms, TE = 100 ms (T2 weighting)

After the second RF pulse (180°), a new signal is formed and is used to produce the image. The 180° RF pulse can be compared with a wall: it reflects the first signal in the form of an echo signal that increases then decreases.[1]

TE is therefore the time between the beginning of the sequence and the middle of the echo.

---

[1] Echo formation. We know that the protons are in phase immediately after excitation (90° RF pulse) (Fig. 3.10.1), and that they progressively lose their phase coherence, since some of them precess faster than others (Fig. 3.10.2; proton speed decreases from *a* to *d*). As mentioned before, this dephasing is caused by two processes: intrinsic T2 difference between tissues, and local Bo inhomogeneities (see p. 13, notes 1 and 2).

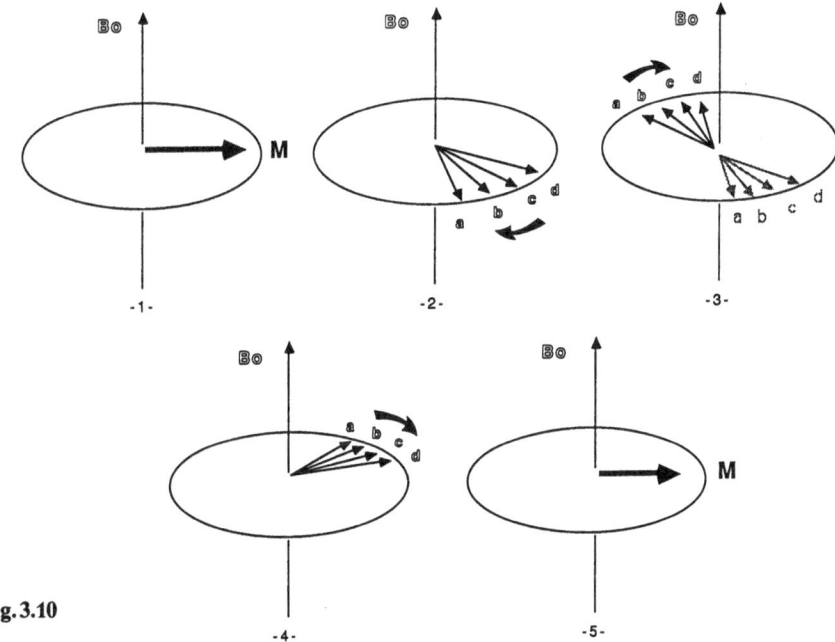

Fig. 3.10

If a 180° pulse is applied at this time, the fastest protons *(a)* are placed *behind* the slowest ones *(d)* (Fig. 3.10.3). But a second and more important effect of the 180° pulse is that it reverses the effect of the local field inhomogeneities on the protons, eventually cancelling them: the artifact associated with nonuniform Bo is corrected. However, the intrinsic T2 effects are of course not cancelled, and continue to act.
As the protons still run at their respective speeds, the fastest catch up on the slowest (Fig. 3.10.4): all protons are soon in phase again, and the M vector is partially restored. The signal obtained at this moment (Fig. 3.10.5) is the "echo" of the original signal in that it is similar but weaker, precisely because of the T2 intrinsic effects that can then be measured.

Spin echo makes it possible to see all three MRI parameters: ρ, T1 and T2. It is the *only* sequence that takes T2 into account, hence its importance for diagnosis.

The image in ρ, T1 and T2 can be weighted by manipulating TR and TE:[1]

TR variations

> short TR: strongly T1-weighted image
> long TR: less T1-weighted image
> In practice, TR ranges from 300 to 2500 ms.

TE variations

> short TE: slightly T2-weighted image
> long TE: strongly T2-weighted image
> In practice, TE ranges from 20 to 120 ms.

As for ρ, it can be enhanced by using very long TR and very short TE: ρ-weighted image.

Table 3.1 summarizes the effect of TR and TE on T1 and T2.

Table 3.1

	Short TR	Long TR
Short TE	T1 image	ρ-T1-(T2) image
Long TE	T1-T2 image	T2 image

---

[1] The influence of TR on T1 weighting may be explained as for partial saturation (see footnote 1, p. 23). Reconsideration of the curves shown previously in Fig. 2.15 makes it possible to understand the effect of TE on T2 weighting (Fig. 3.9).

Changing TE means altering the stage of T2 relaxation at which the image is obtained:

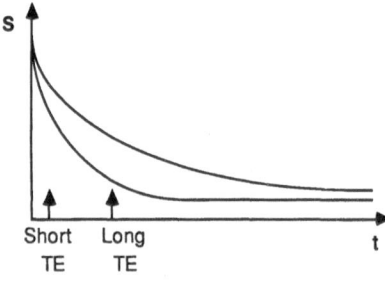

Fig. 3.9

If a short TE is chosen, the image is taken at a time when T2 differences have not yet appeared. If TE is long, the image may be highly T2-weighted.

Multiple Spin Echo

Structure

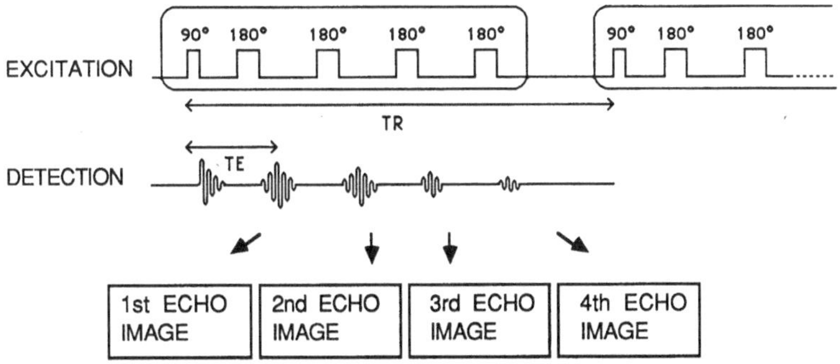

Fig. 3.11

Excitation: Each sequence is made of one 90° RF pulse followed by a variable number of 180° RF pulses (up to eight, generally two or four). As far as time intervals are concerned, we therefore find:

TR between two sequences.

TE: the first echo comes at TE1, the second echo after a time TE2 which is longer, etc.

Detection: For the *same slice,* the machine therefore generates an image of the first echo, then one of the second echo, etc.

Notice that the signal decays progressively as the distance from the 90° pulse increases: an image of the fourth echo always has a lower signal-to-noise ratio than that of the first echo.

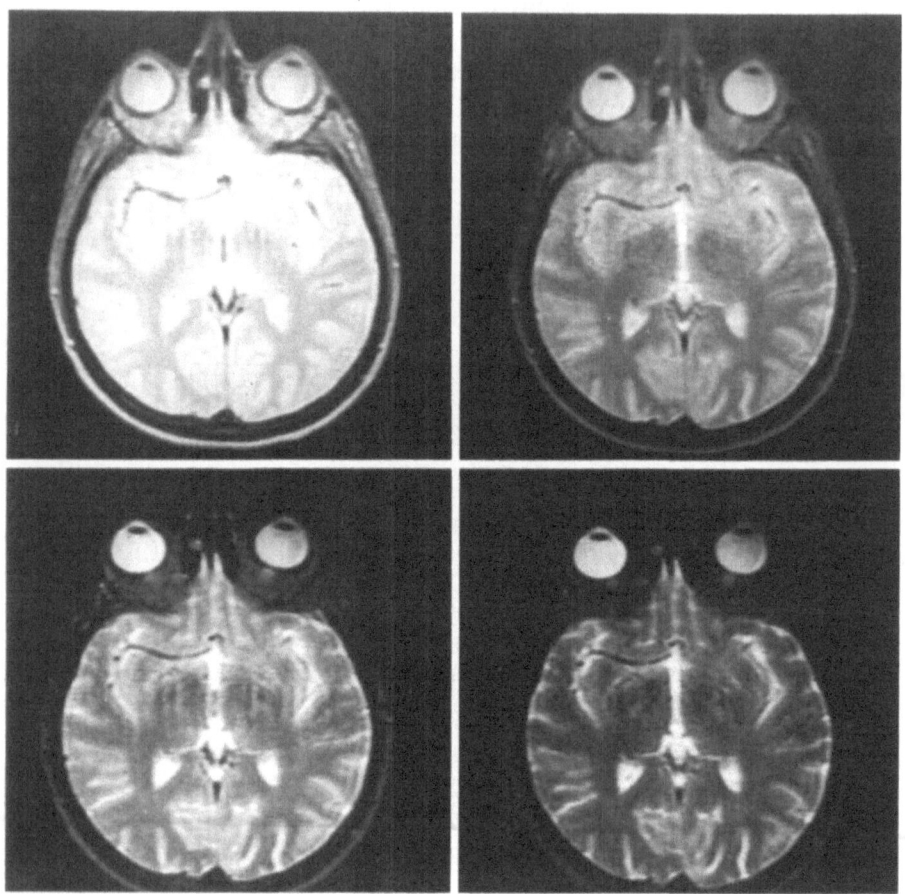

Fig. 3.12. Axial sections of the brain. TR = 2500 ms, TE = 25 ms; four symmetric echoes

Like spin echo, multiple spin echo is based on all three MR parameters: ρ, T1 and T2. It has the advantage of allowing for progressive enhancement of T2 weighting of the image in the later echoes[1]. Sequences of more than four echoes are rarely of practical use because of the signal decay due to T2 relaxation effects.

Two types of echoes can be used:

Symmetric echoes (for example: TE = 25 ms, giving an image of the second echo at 50 ms, of the third echo at 75 ms, etc.)

Asymmetric echoes (for example: TE = 30 ms for the first echo, TE = 100 ms for the second echo)

---

[1] In this case, too, the T2 relaxation curve makes it possible to represent what occurs when multiple spin echo is used (Fig. 3.13).

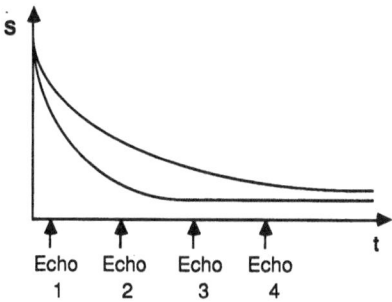

Fig. 3.13

When several echoes are programmed, several "photographs" of relaxation are taken successively. The later the echo, the higher the contrast between two kinds of tissue will be. However, very long TE produces weak signals for all kinds of tissue studied.

Inversion Recovery

Structure

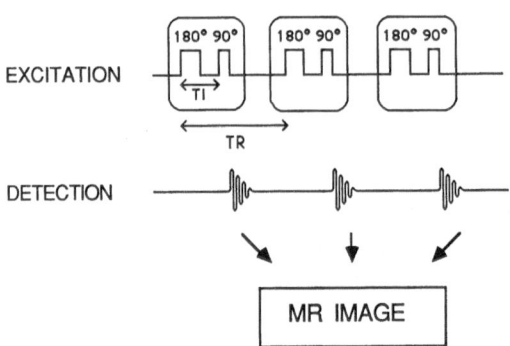

EXCITATION

180° 90° | 180° 90° | 180° 90°

TI

TR

DETECTION

MR IMAGE

Fig. 3.14

Excitation: Each pulse sequence includes two RF pulses, 180° then 90°. Therefore there are two time intervals:

TR between two sequences.

TI (inversion time) between the 180° pulse and the 90° pulse within the same sequence. The term "inversion time" comes from the fact that each sequence begins with an inversion of the M vector that flips 180° relative to its equilibrium position.

Detection: The 180° pulse does not generate a signal the machine can detect. The signal appears only after the 90° pulse.

Use

Inversion recovery makes it possible to represent two of the three MR parameters: ρ and T1. The relative proportions of ρ and T1 can be controlled using two acquisition parameters: TR and TI. In practice, inversion recovery is used to obtain T1-weighted images (Same reasons as for partial saturation).

Question: Why was inversion recovery created when the imaging of ρ and T1 was already possible with partial saturation?

Answer: Inversion recovery allows for better T1 contrast than partial saturation. In fact, when the protons undergo the initial 180° flip (instead of 90°), the recovery of the protons in the different tissues is better differentiated. (It is easier to compare the performance of cars in a 100-km race than in a 50-km race) (Fig. 3.16).

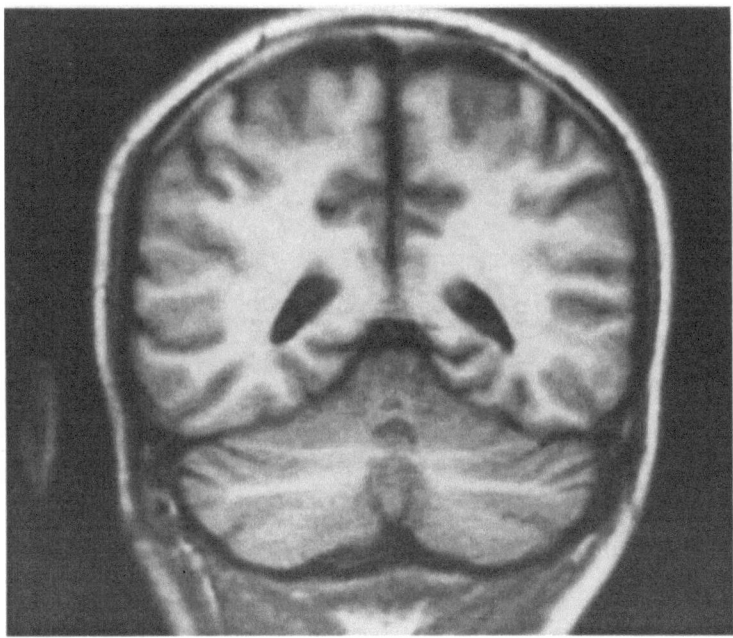

Fig. 3.15. Frontal section of the brain through the occipital horns of the lateral ventricles and the cerebellum. TR = 1500 ms, TI = 600 ms. Note the very good contrast between white and gray matter

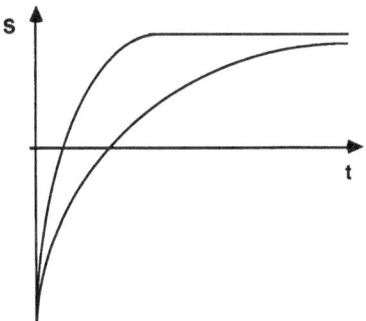

Fig. 3.16

Inversion recovery has one drawback in that it (usually) does not allow one to obtain T2-weighted images. Moreover, the spin echo sequence allows for quite satisfactory T1-weighted imaging. For those reasons, many centers use spin echo almost exclusively.

Note. For technical reasons, all MRI sequences end with an echo. This is true for inversion recovery, as well as for partial saturation. Adding an 180° RF pulse is equivalent to transforming these sequences into a spin echo sequence, but with significant T1 weighting, since very short TE ($\leqslant 20$ ms) are used for these two pulse sequences, thus making them insensitive to T2.

Summary

Pulse sequences are the "tools" enabling protons excitation. There are several types of sequences (according to the order of the RF pulses). Each type can be modified by setting the *time intervals* appropriately:

  TR: repetition time
  TE: echo time
  TI: inversion time

Pulse sequences and time intervals are therefore the *acquisition parameters* (or machine parameters).

Remember that ρ, T1 and T2 are characteristics of the tissue. As such, they are referred to as *tissue parameters*.

We know that an MR image is a combination of ρ, T1 and T2. Altering the acquisition parameters makes it possible to manipulate the weight of each tissue parameter in the image (Fig. 3.17).

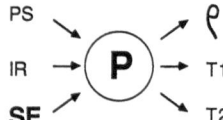

Fig. 3.17

Fast Imaging

Imaging time is relatively long in the sequences we have just described (see p.64). For that reason, sequences called "fast imaging", allowing for imaging times only one-tenth as long as usual or even shorter, have appeared. Of the various methods used, we will describe the commonly used procedure called "gradient reversal echo."

Structure

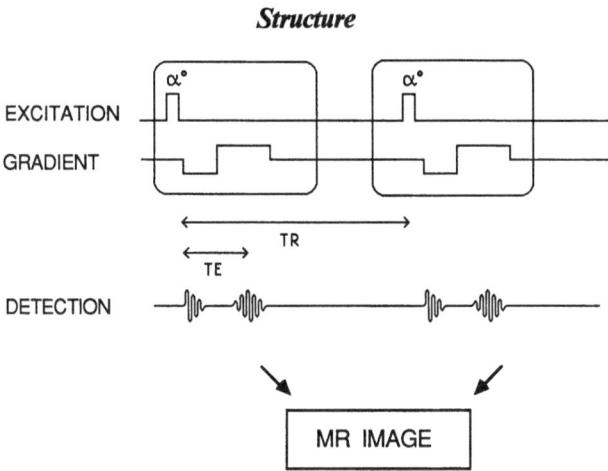

Fig. 3.18

Excitation: Each sequence includes only one pulse causing the M vector to rotate to a chosen angle ($\alpha°$ angle) ranging from 5° to 90°.

Instead of creating an echo (which is necessary, see p.31) by means of a 180° RF pulse, a technological trick is resorted to: gradient reversal (see Appendix 2).

Three machine parameters can be described:

    TR: repetition time elapsing between two sequences
    TE: echo time
    $\alpha°$: angle of M vector flip in relation to Bo

Detection: As in spin echo, the MR image is generated using only the echo signal.

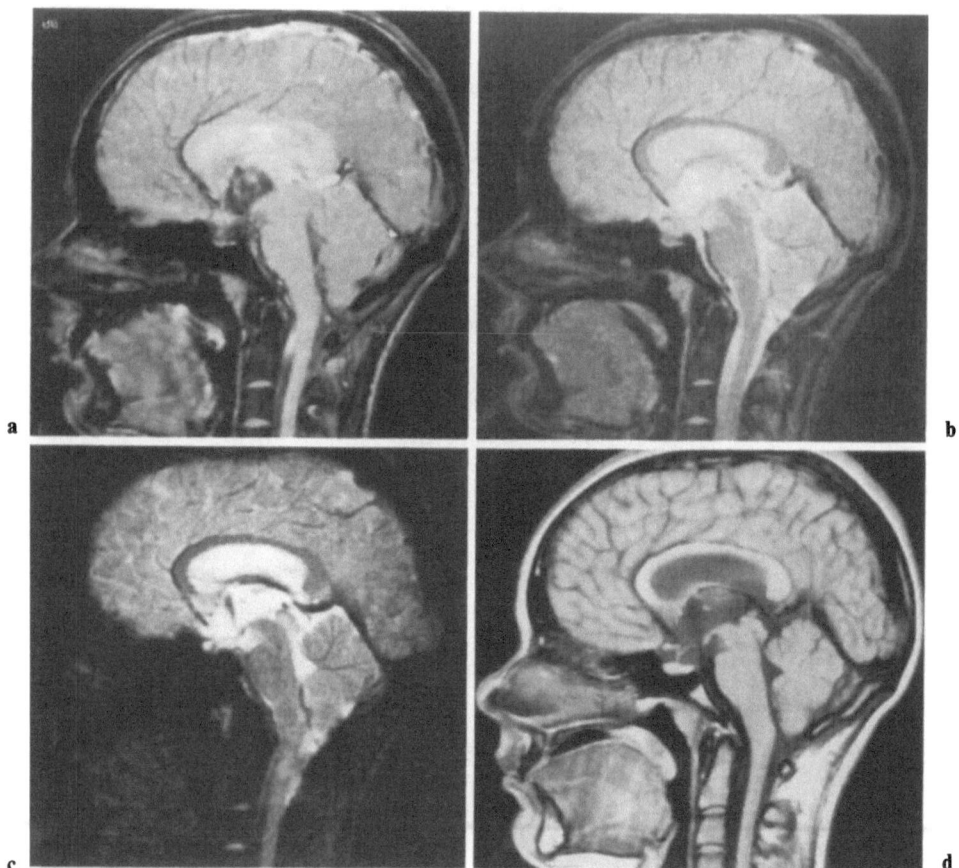

Fig. 3.19 a–d. Supratentorial ventricular enlargement consecutive to stenosis of the cerebral aqueduct. Fast imaging. **a** T1 weighting (TR = 200 ms, TE = 12 ms, $\alpha^\circ = 90^\circ$). **b** ρ weighting (TR = 200 ms, TE = 12 ms, $\alpha^\circ = 10^\circ$). **c** T2 weighting (TR = 200 ms, TE = 50 ms, $\alpha^\circ = 10^\circ$). **d** For comparison, same section in spin echo, T1 weighting (TR = 500 ms, TE = 20 ms)

Like spin echo, fast imaging makes it possible to visualize ρ, T1 and T2. The image can be weighted by adjusting all three acquisition parameters: TR, TE and $\alpha°$ (Table 3.2).

Table 3.2

	T1-weighted	T2-weighted		ρ-weighted
		*	**	
TR (ms)	200–400	20–50	200–400	200–400
TE (ms)	12–15	12–15	30–60	12–15
$\alpha°$ (deg.)	45–90	30–60	5–20	5–20

* Some T2 weighting
** Heavily T2 weighting
Wehrli F. (1987) Introduction to Fast-Scan Magnetic Resonance, General Electric.

The use of very short TR is the factor actually permitting considerable reduction of imaging time. However, shortening TR has the drawback of decreasing the signal strength, and thereby reducing image quality (see Fig. 3.7).
Fast imaging has three main advantages (which we shall come back to later):

Shorter scanning times (including the ability to get rapid images for localization, "scout views")
Images taken with the patient holding his breath
Sequences more sensitive to flow effects (blood vessels and cerebrospinal fluid)

Fast imaging sequences thus represent a new and important MR procedure (Fig. 3.20).

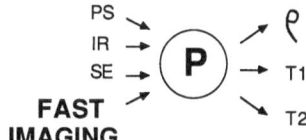

Fig. 3.20

35

Chapter 4 Contribution to Diagnosis

Any imaging technique aims at answering two questions:

$$\left.\begin{array}{l}\textit{Morphology}\\\textit{Nature}\end{array}\right\}\quad \text{of the pathological process}$$

MRI brings new answers to these questions.

Morphological Diagnosis

Location?
Size?
Shape?
Extent?
Relations?
etc.

In order to diagnose a pathological process and to assess its morphological characteristics, the physician performing a MRI examination must make two decisions:

(1) *Which imaging plane?*
(2) *Which pulse sequence?*

Choice of Imaging Plane

MRI makes it possible to select slices directly in any spatial direction. In practice, the three orthogonal section planes are used:

Axial
Sagittal
Coronal

It is now possible to perform oblique imaging with most MR machines.

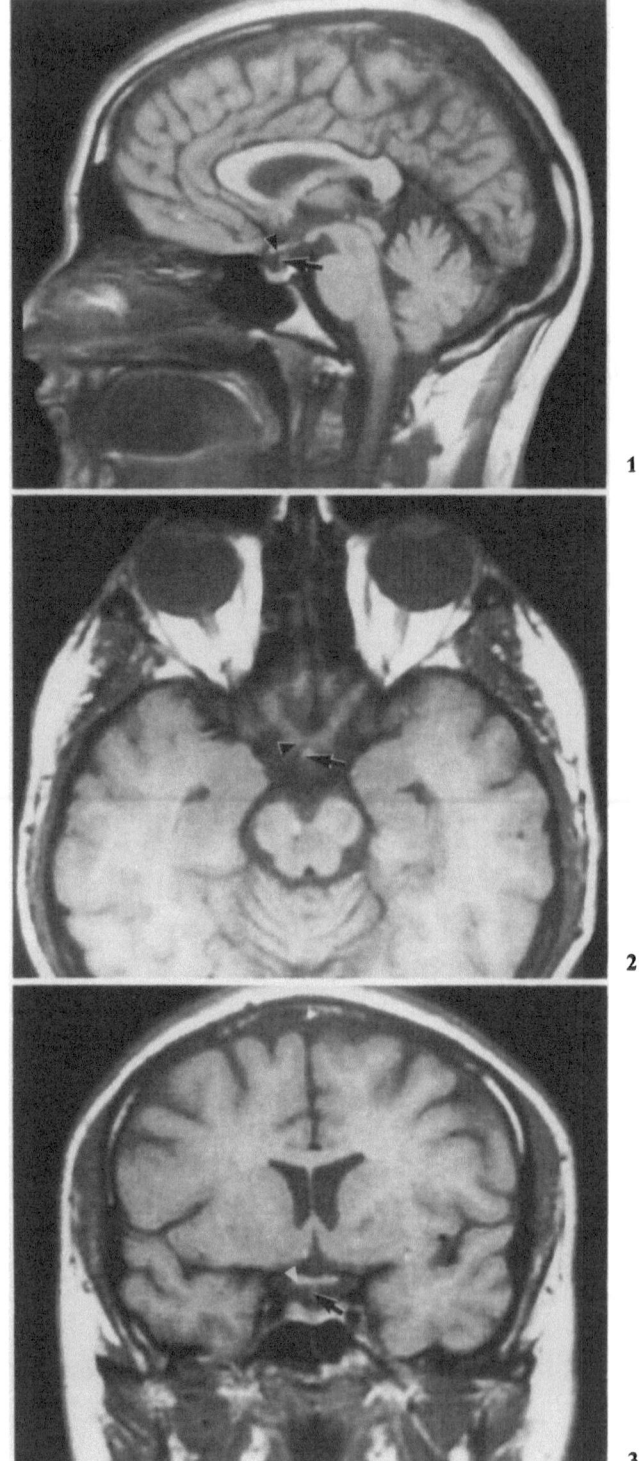

Fig. 4.1a

38

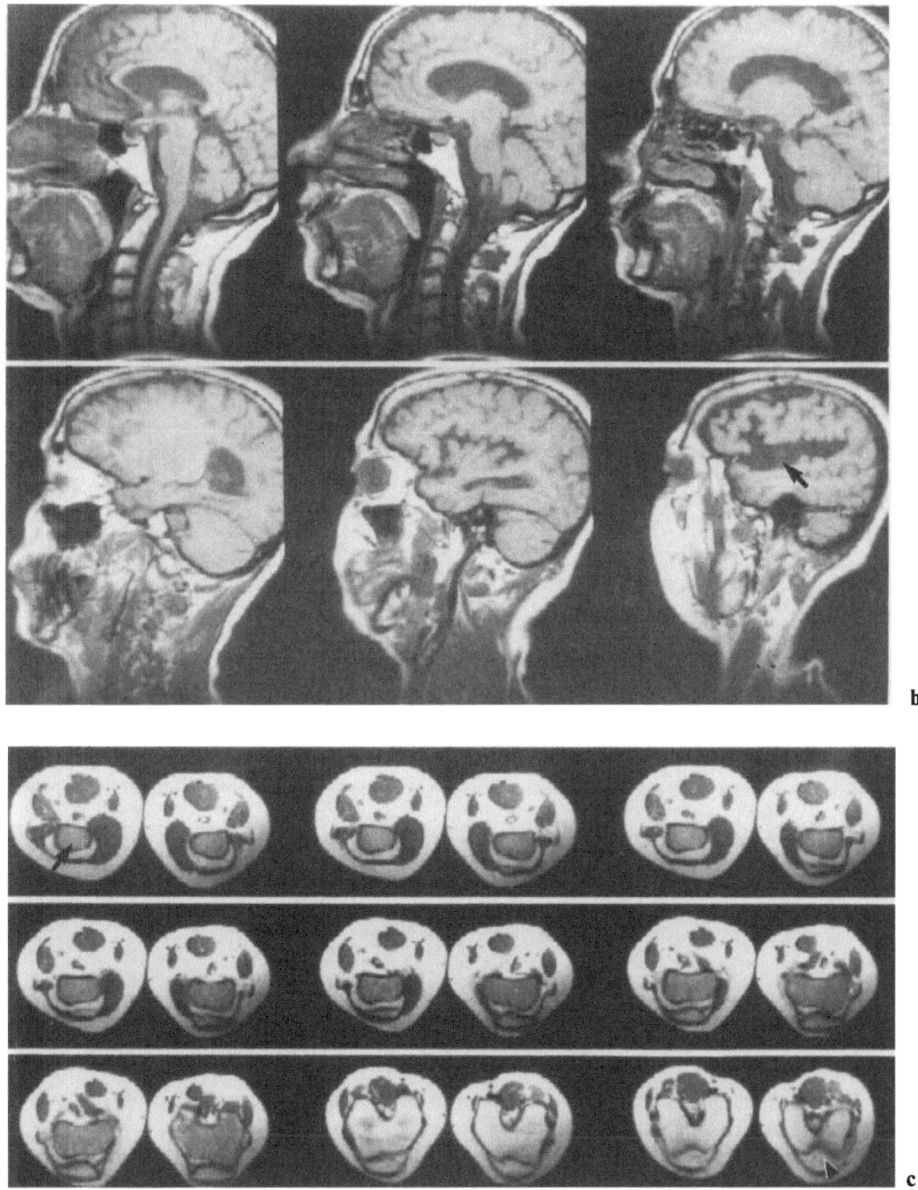

b

c

Fig. 4.1. a1–a3. Sagittal, axial and coronal sections at the level of the optic chiasma (▶) and the pituitary stalk (➔). **b** Sagittal sections of the brain and of the facial structures from the mid-sagittal plane *(top left)* to the sylvian fissure *(bottom right)*. Note major cortical atrophy (➔). **c** Axial section across the lower limbs, from the medial part of the femoral diaphysis (➔) *(top left)* to the patellae (▶) and the femoral condyles *(bottom right)*

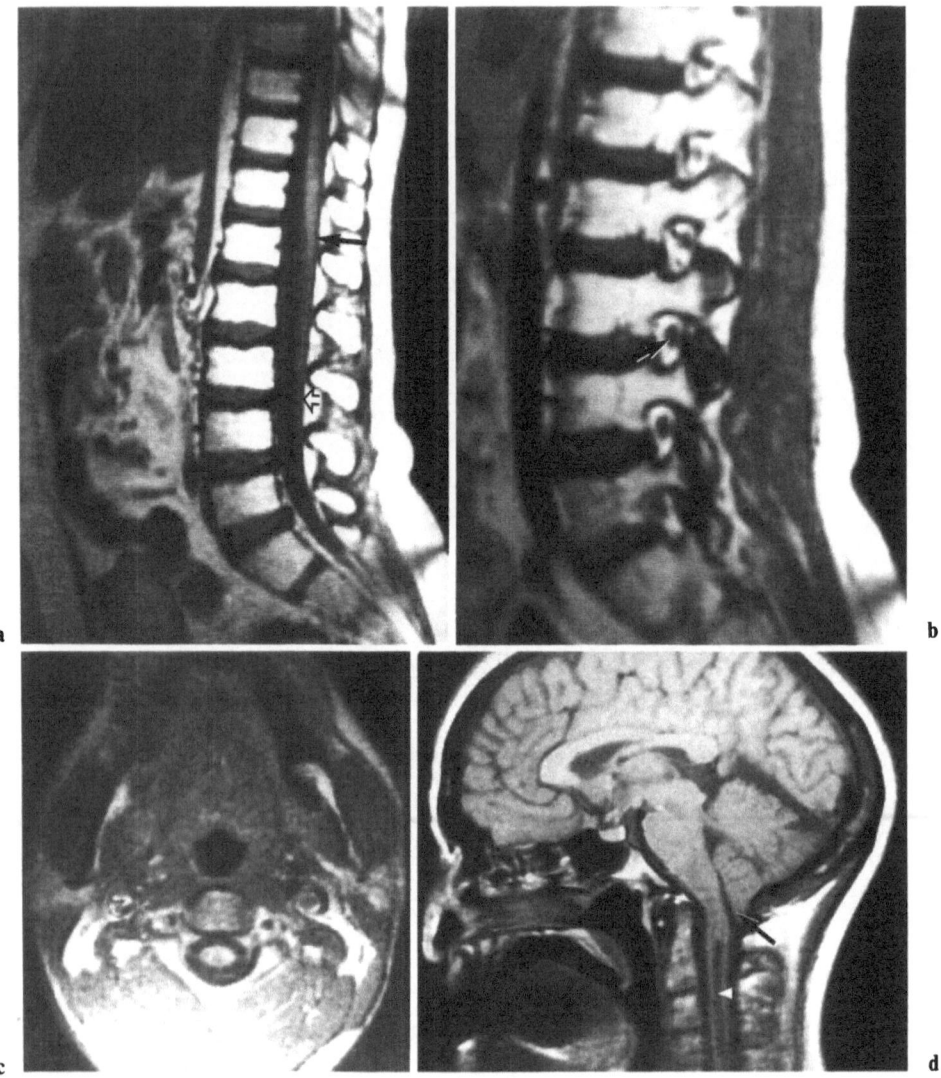

Fig. 4.2 a–d. **a** Midsagittal section of the lower dorsal and lumbosacral spine. The cord ends at L1 (➔) and is followed by the filum terminale that can be identified down to L3–L4 (⊰), **b** Parasagittal section of the spine at the level of the intervertebral foramina. The neurovascular bundle can be identified (➔) in its fatty environment. **c** Axial section of the upper cervical cord. **d** Sagittal section across the craniocervical junction. The tonsil of the cerebellum (➔) lies under the foramen magnum, indicating a Chiari malformation. There is also a cervical syringomyelia (▶).

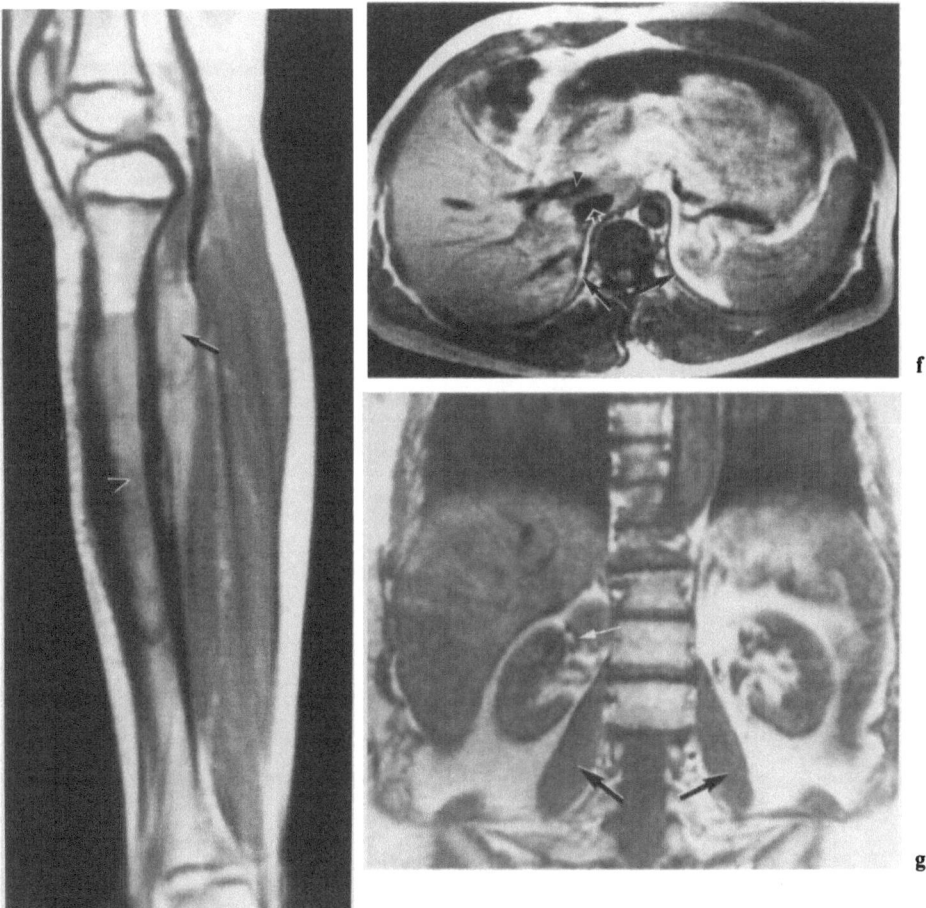

Fig. 4.2 e–g. **e** Sagittal section of the leg. Ewing's sarcoma at tibial level. The expansion of the sarcoma can be assessed in the bone (▶). Its extension in soft tissue is also clearly depicted (➔). **f** Axial section of the abdomen across the right lobe of the liver, the spleen, the aorta, the crus of the diaphragm (➔), the inferior vena cava (↦) and the portal vein (▶). **g** Coronal section of the abdomen across the kidneys and the psoas muscles (➔). A surgical scar can be identified at the upper part of the right kidney (➔).

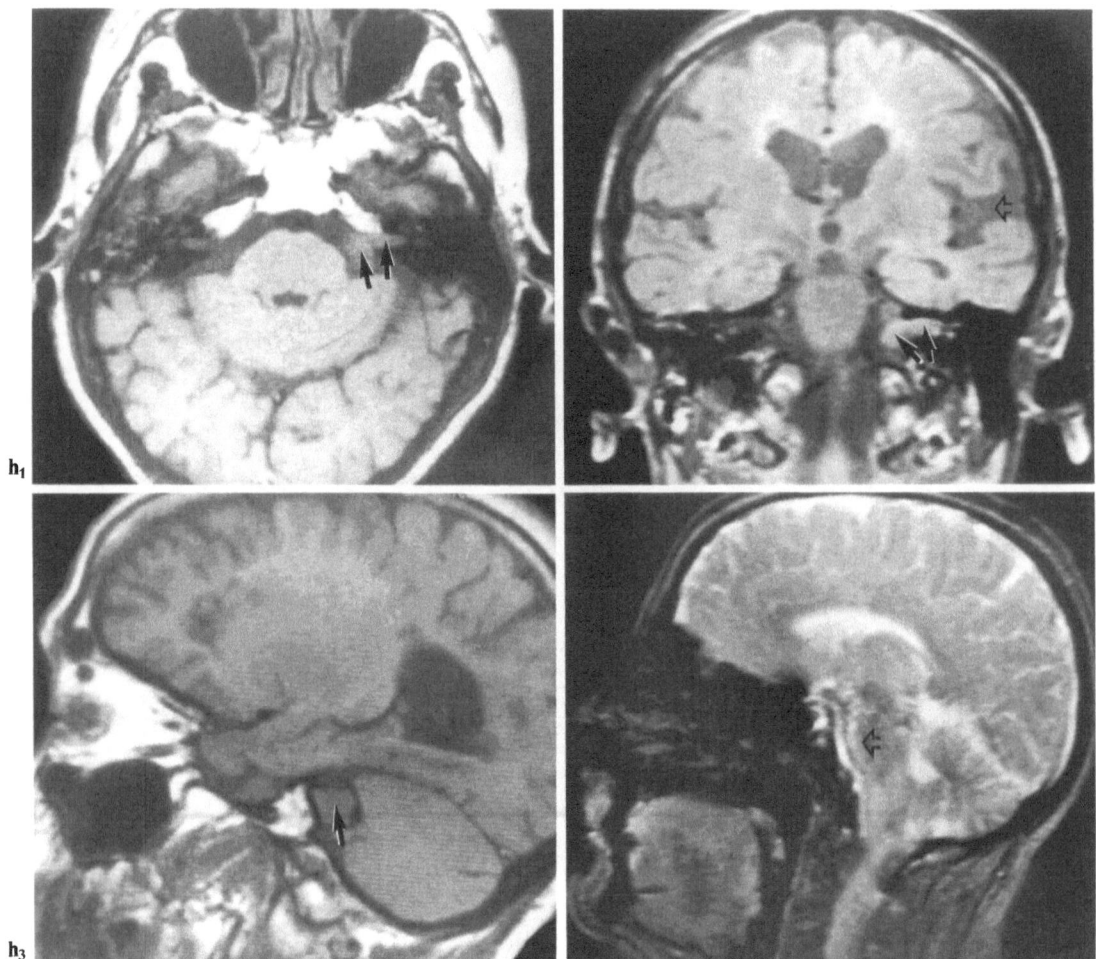

Fig. 4.2 h–i. **h1–h3** Axial, coronal and left parasagittal sections across the left cerebellopontine angle. An acoustic neurinoma is depicted inside and outside the internal auditory canal (→). Notice the significant cortical atrophy that is clearly visible at the level of the left sylvian fissure in the coronal plane (↔). **i** Midsagittal section of the brain. Three-second scout view (fast imaging). Despite relatively poor definition, it is already possible to identify a space-occupying lesion in the brain stem (↔)

Moreover, MRI generates a series of slices in the chosen plane:[1]

Top ↔ bottom (axial plane)
Right ↔ left (sagittal plane)
Anterior ↔ posterior (coronal plane).

In practice, the choice of imaging planes, i.e., the number of planes and their programming order, depends on the following (Fig. 4.1, 4.2):

Anatomy. The examination of the spinal cord begins with sagittal sections. The second set is usually composed of axial slices. The coronal plane is seldom used because of the physiological curvatures of the spine in the sagittal plane.
For the abdominal organs (liver, spleen, pancreas, kidneys, adrenals) and the genitopelvic organs, two planes are often sufficient.

Pathology. An abnormality in the craniocervical junction, such as a Chiari malformation, can be imaged best in the sagittal plane.
The extent of a tumor in a long bone will be demonstrated by sections in a plane parallel to the diaphysis (coronal or sagittal).
Preoperative brain workup is an indication for assessment in all three orthogonal planes, in order to give the surgeon the maximal number of anatomical indications.

Finally, it should be remembered that fast imaging makes it possible to perform scout views within seconds.

Choice of Pulse Sequence

It is essential to have at least one T1-weighted and one T2-weighted sequence for each examination.
Why? Let us study the (fictive) case of a tumor developing in a given tissue A. As we have seen, each kind of tissue is characterized by its relaxation times T1 and T2 (ms).

	T1	T2
Tumor	800	50
Tissue A	400	50
Contrast	+	0

---

[1] Computed tomography (CT) only allows for direct axial imaging. Coronal or sagittal images obtained with last generation systems are reformatted from axial sections: their resolution is therefore noticeably lower.

For details on the technical aspects of slice selection, see Appendix 2.

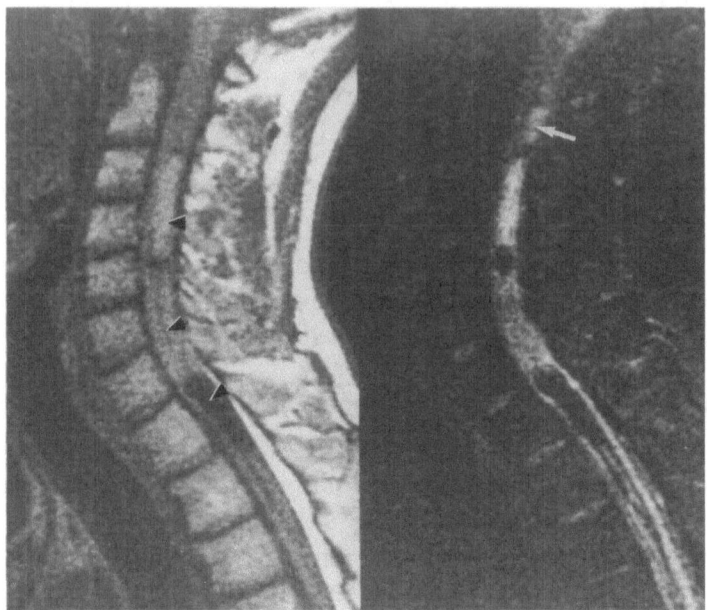

Fig. 4.3. Sagittal sections of the cervicodorsal spine. Large spinal cord astrocytoma (▶). The T2-weighted sequence *(right)* shows that the upper extent of the lesion is one vertebral level higher (➡) than was evident with the T1-weighted sequence *(left)*

A T2-weighted image shows no contrast between the tumor and tissue A, since they have the same T2. A T1-weighted image, however, will enhance the tumor.

Suppose now that the tissue A is surrounded by another tissue B with its own T1 and T2 (ms)

	T1	T2
Tumor	800	50
Tissue B	800	100
Contrast	0	+

The T2-weighted sequence will make it possible to assess the extent of the pathological process in tissue B.

Therefore, each of the two sequences has played a part in establishing the diagnosis.

Thus, morphological diagnosis supposes that slices be made in at least two, at best three, spatial planes with at least one T1-weighted sequence and one T2-weighted sequence. However, we shall see (p. 64) that T1-weighted images

44

are obtained more rapidly than T2-weighted ones. Moreover, we know that T2-weighted images have a lower signal-to-noise ratio and sometimes poor spatial resolution. For these two reasons, T1-weighted sequences alone are sometimes considered as "morphological" sequences that should always be performed as a first step.

In any case, characterization of pathological processes can only be approached on the basis of a combination of T1-weighted and T2-weighted images.

Nature of the Pathological Process

Assessing the nature of the pathological process under study requires interpretation of the very parameters making up the image, especially relaxation times. Whereas in CT there is "hypo- or hyperdensities," in MRI one speaks of "hypo- or hyperintense signal" in T1- or T2-weighted images and tries to determine the relation between a type of signal in a precise sequence and a kind of tissue.

Thus a double question has to be asked:

Given the signal of a tissue, can its T1 and T2 be assessed?
Given the T1 and T2 of a tissue, can its nature be determined?

$$\text{T1/T2} \overset{?}{\longleftrightarrow} \text{Tissue}$$

In other words, does MRI make it possible to characterize tissues precisely? There is no definitive answer to this question; even though the hopes aroused in the early days of MRI do not seem to have been fulfilled, the method has nevertheless brought a number of assets, which we will now examine.

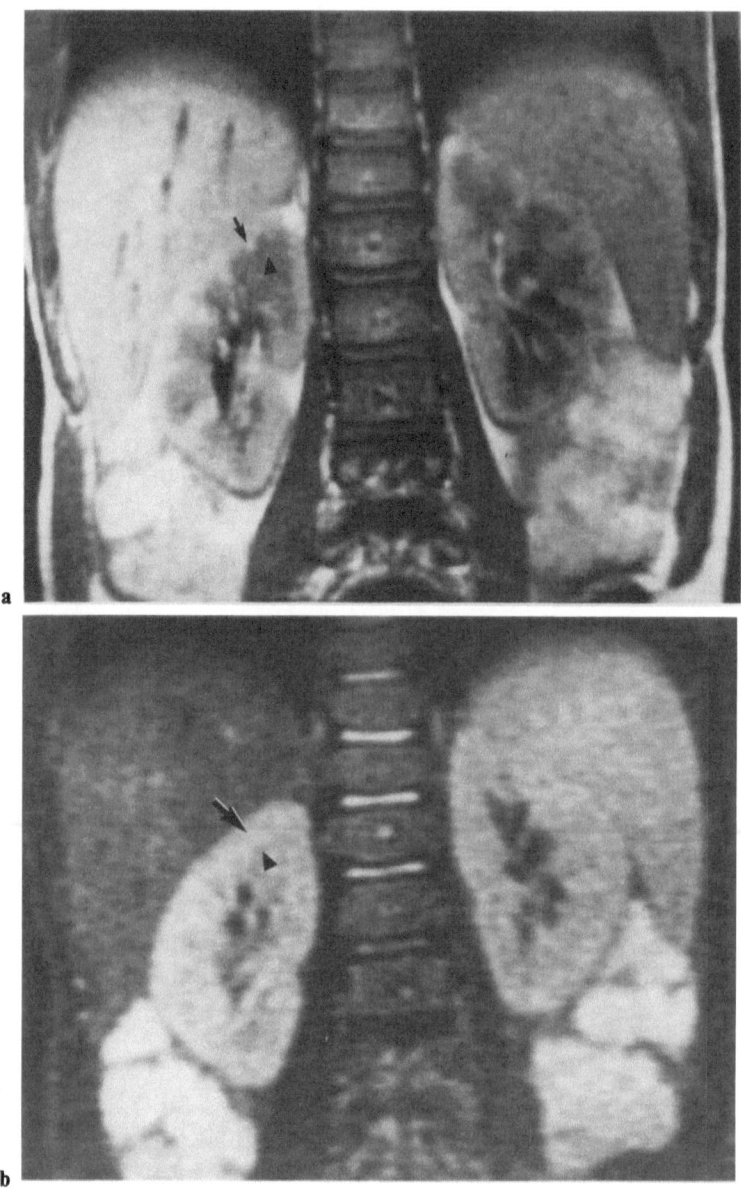

Fig. 4.4a, b. Coronal sections across the kidneys, the liver, the spleen and the spine. **a** T1 weighting; **b** T2 weighting. The medulla of the kidney (▶) appears hypointense in T1 and hyperintense in T2, whereas the cortex (→) shows T1 hyperintensity and T2 hypointensity

Hypointense, Hyperintense Signal (Fig. 4.4 a, b)

We know that when excited protons return to equilibrium – when they relax – they induce a signal and that all signals combine to generate the MR image.

Whatever relaxation time (T1 or T2) is considered:

> If the emitted signal is *low* it is called *hypo*intense and represented in *black*
> If the emitted signal is *high* it is called *hyper*intense and represented in *white*

Interpretation Rules for Spin Echo

The rules of interpretation for spin echo are deduced from equations which make it possible to determine the relaxation times from the intensity of the signals.

For T1-weighted images:

> Hyposignal = tissue with long T1
> Hypersignal = tissue with short T1

For T2-weighted images:

> Hyposignal = tissue with short T2
> Hypersignal = tissue with long T2

The inversion in interpretation rules for T1 and T2 images is logical and can be understood if relaxation curves are considered (Fig. 4.5 a, b).

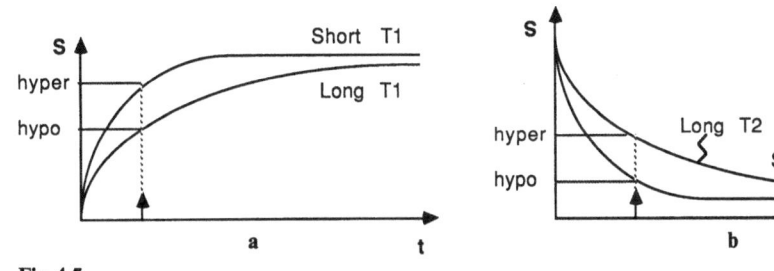

Fig. 4.5

T1 and T2 Characteristics of Body Tissues (Fig. 4.6)

In MRI, soft tissues are classified into three categories:

> Fats (subcutaneous fat, abdominal fat, etc.)
> "Pure" liquids (CSF, urine, etc.)
> "Impure" liquids (i.e., parenchymas: liver, brain, kidneys, etc.)

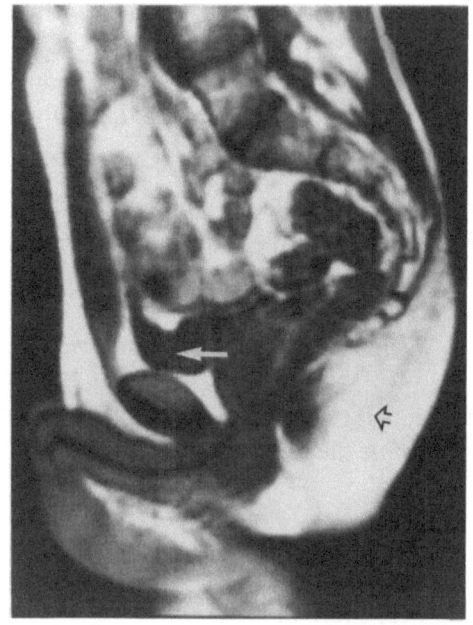

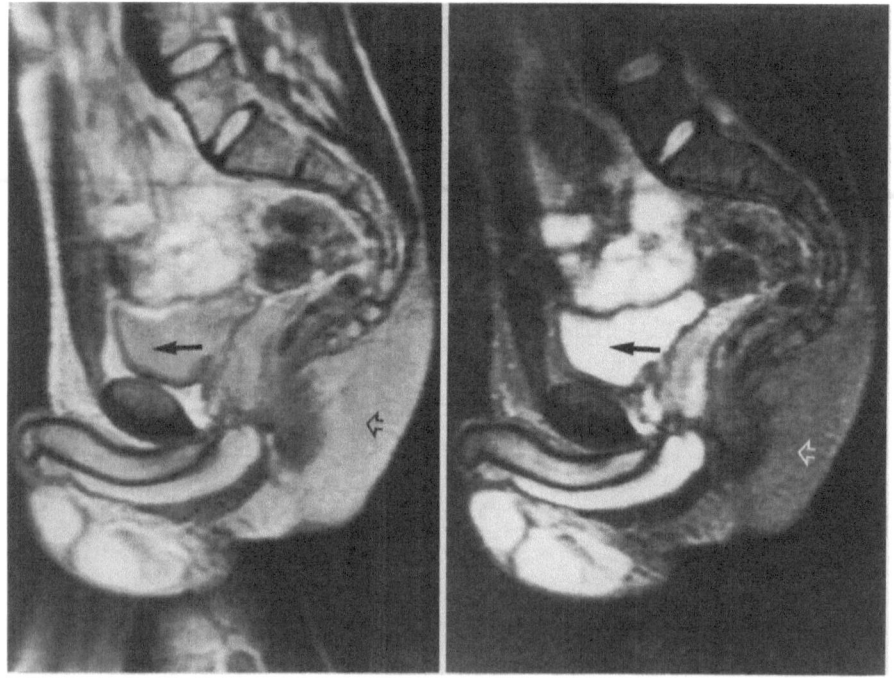

Fig. 4.6a–c. Sagittal sections of a male pelvis. Notice the signal changes in urine (→) and fat (⇗). Water and fat are isointense in **b** (signal crossing area). **a** T1-weighted sequence (TR = 600 ms, TE = 20 ms). **b** mixed ρ-T1-(T2)-weighted sequence (TR = 2000 ms, TE = 30 ms). **c** T2-weighted sequence (TR = 2000 ms, TE = 100 ms)

In T1, these three types of tissue are distributed as follows:

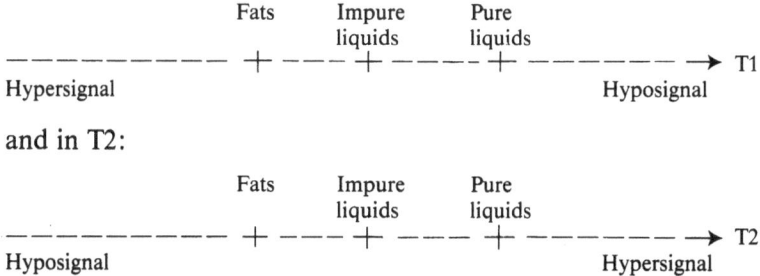

and in T2:

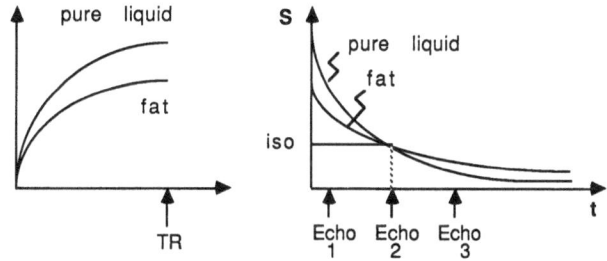

This logical distribution of the three tissue types along the T1 and T2 signal scales ensues from the fact that fat has short T1 and T2 and water long T1 and T2, parenchymas being intermediate (see p. 11 and 13).

Signal Crossing (Fig. 4.6)

In T1 and T2 distribution diagrams, we can see that CSF (or urine) produces a hypointense signal in a T1-weighted sequence and a hyperintense signal in a T2-weighted sequence. Since fat reacts in the opposite way, there has to be sequences in which water and fat have the same signal *(isosignal)*. In effect, this occurs in mixed ρ-T1-(T2) sequence.

Figure 4.7 gives an example of a mixed sequence with short TR and three echoes:

Fig. 4.7

The choice of a short TR enhances the T1 contrast between fats and pure liquids, and on the T2 decay curve, each tissue starts at a different level. But, since fats are characterized by a short T2 and pure liquids by a long T2, there is a crossing point between the two curves where the two substances show an isointense signal; contrast has reversed between the first and the third echo.

Signal crossing does not occur in all kinds of tissue. Some substances (like air or cortical bone) keep the same signal in T1 and in T2 images, and no crossing occurs in them.

49

Air and Cortical Bone (Fig. 4.8)

Air, cortical bone, and dense calcifications appear as hypointense areas *whatever sequence is used*.
This constant hyposignal is essentially caused by the very low proton density (and therefore the small number or lack of protons to be excited) of these substances.

Quantitative Analysis (Fig. 4.9)

So far we have described tissue relaxation times in semiquantitative terms (longer or shorter T1 and T2).

Is it possible to calculate T1 and T2 reliably?
Can a given tissue in a given state be allotted precise values for T1 and T2?
Above all, can two tissues be distinguished on this basis?

At the current state of the art, the answers to these questions are as follows:

It is possible to calculate T1 and T2 (and the density of protons) for a given organ using different TRs and TEs for the same slice. On the basis of these values, so-called synthetic images can be generated: these may be T1 or T2 maps, in which each point, each picture element, represents the T1 (or T2) calculated by the machine, or may be synthetic TR/TE images, where the calculated T1 and T2 values are used to reconstruct the images of a sequence not performed during patient examination.
However, such calculations are beset by errors, arising mainly from the MR apparatus itself, but also, to a minor degree, from other MRI factors influencing the image (diffusion, flow, etc.). Motion also often alters the quality of measurements.

Even when the calculation is reliable, there is a significant margin of error in the calculated values. Moreover, many healthy tissues have similar relaxation times and a pathological condition does not always involve major alterations (increase or decrease) of relaxation times. "Pathological" identification of a tissue using the calculated T1 and T2 values is therefore usually not possible.

Since the calculated T1 and T2 values frequently *overlap,* it is often not possible to discriminate between two soft tissues in a given individual.

Lastly, relaxation times change with the intensity of the magnetic field Bo (in particular, T1 increases with increasing Bo). For this reason, the intensity of the field used must always be specified when mentioning calculated T1 and T2 values.

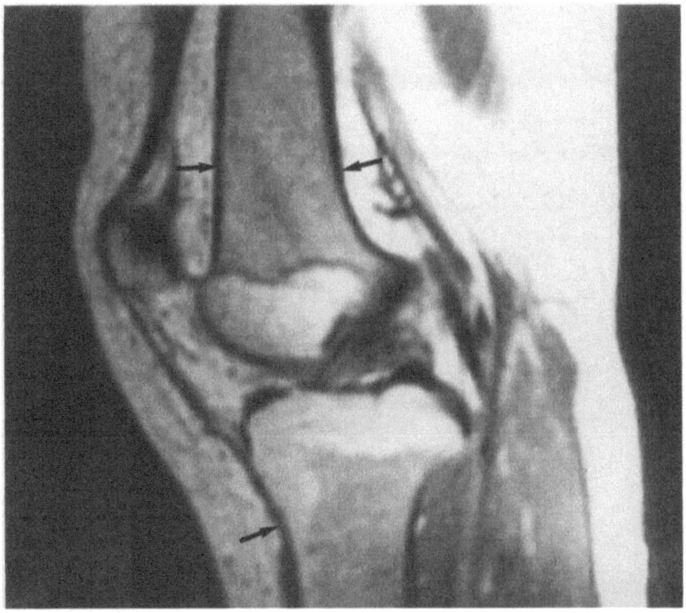

a

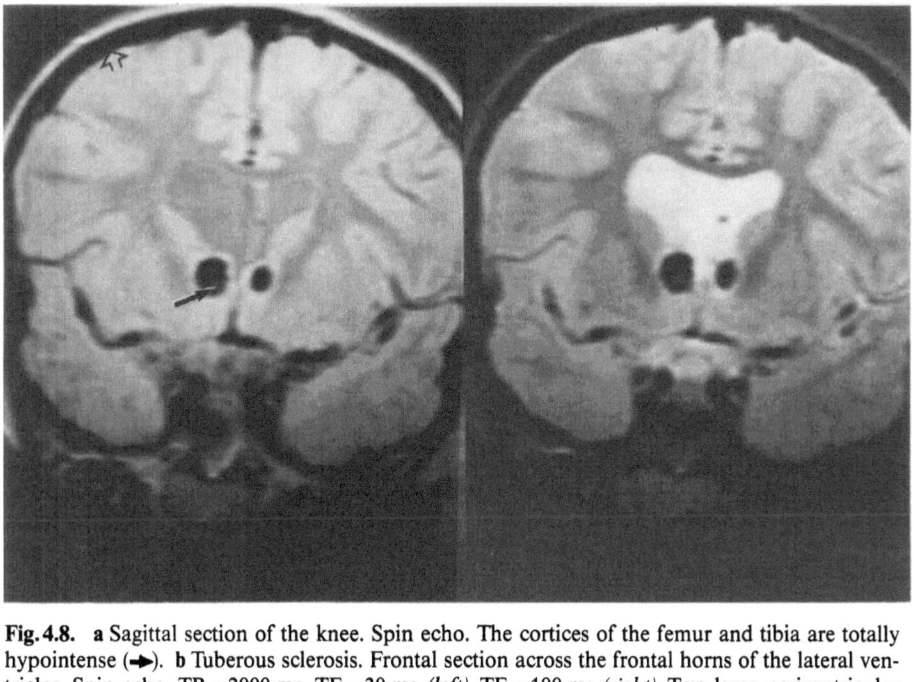

b c

Fig. 4.8. **a** Sagittal section of the knee. Spin echo. The cortices of the femur and tibia are totally hypointense (➔). **b** Tuberous sclerosis. Frontal section across the frontal horns of the lateral ventricles. Spin echo. TR = 2000 ms, TE = 30 ms *(left)*, TE = 100 ms *(right)*. Two large periventricular calcified areas show marked hypointensity on both echo images (➔). Also note the hypointensity of the cranial vault (⇨)

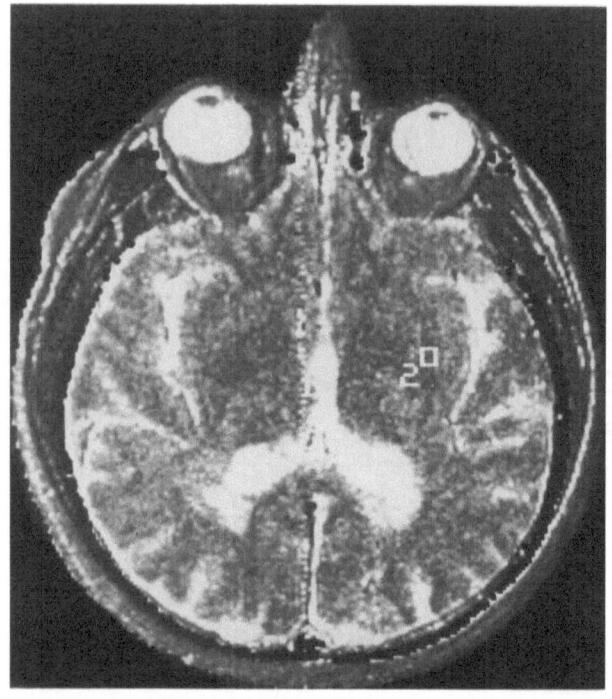

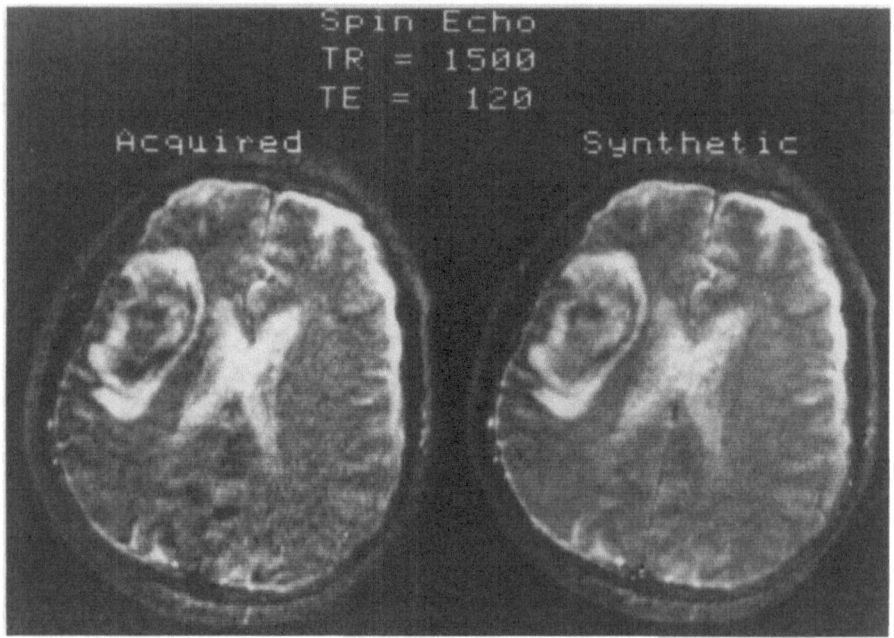

Fig. 4.9. a Axial section of the brain. Calculated T2 map. **b** Axial section of the brain. *Right:* synthetic image simulating a T2-weighted sequence and calculated with values taken from other sequences. *Left:* comparison with the actually performed T2-weighted sequence

All in all, quantitative analysis does not yet constitute a key element of MRI diagnosis.

Thus, determining the nature of a pathological process is both the most interesting and the most difficult aspect of diagnosis.[1] In practice, it should not be attempted without the assistance of history-taking and other additional investigations. Experience will show to what extent MRI speeds diagnosis.

In summary: MRI is an *extremely sensitive* imaging technique, with its multi-section capability and excellent T1 and T2 soft tissue contrast. However, it has an important drawback: its relatively *poor specificity* (T1 [and T2] values overlap).

---

[1] We have given an intentionally simplified description of this process. The exercises at the end of the book will allow readers to test their expertise and will introduce them to two additional factors: flow (Exercise 6) and paramagnetic substances (Exercise 8).

Chapter 5   MR Examination Procedure

Contraindications and Safety Considerations

MR has no known adverse effects on the body. However, some *contraindications* to the use of a very intense magnetic field should be absolutely respected:

Pacemakers, electrical neurostimulators.

Ferromagnetic implants likely to be displaced by the magnetic field (intracranial vascular clips, metallic foreign bodies in soft tissues, etc.)

Some metallic implants (stainless steel dental hardware, hip prosthesis, Harrington rod, etc.), are not contraindications for MR, but cause image artifacts, that are more limited, however, than in CT (see Appendix 1).

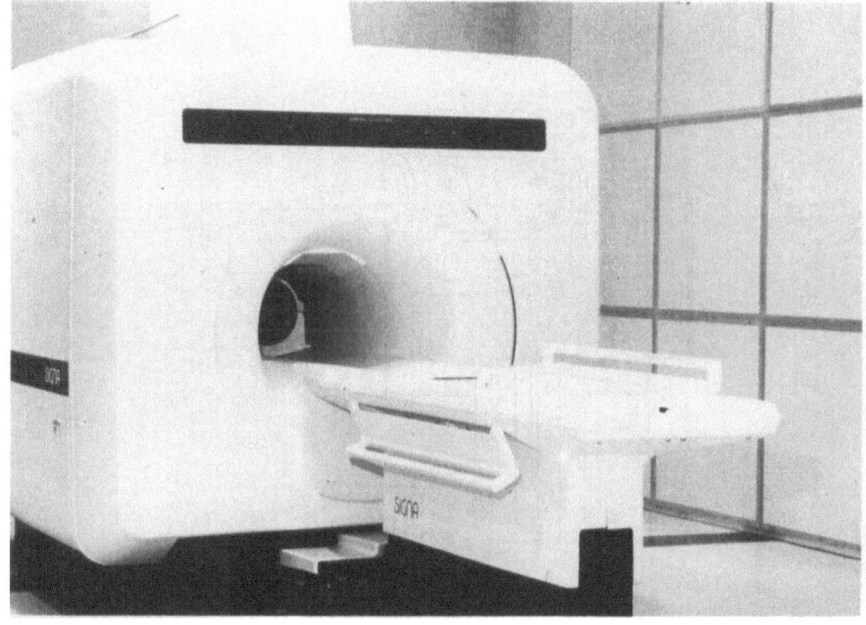

Fig. 5.1

MR has not been proved to have no adverse effects on fetuses, and some teams avoid using it in pregnant women.

Claustrophobia, despite the fact the patient lies in a confined space, is rarely a serious problem, given good patient management.

Children and agitated patients should be sedated before examination.

Lastly, the patient should remove any metallic object (keys, coins, jewels, hair-pins, removable dental bridgework, etc.) before entering the machine.

The MR Machine (Fig. 5.1)

A mobile bed facilitates insertion of the patient into the machine. The area to be studied is positioned at the center of the magnet.

The MR System (Fig. 5.2)

The magnet (1) is a key element of the MR apparatus. It is integrated into a system which also includes:

(2) A radiofrequency emission/reception coil
(3) Gradient coils (see Appendix 2)
(4) Data collection and processing systems
(5) Power supplies
(6) A control and display console

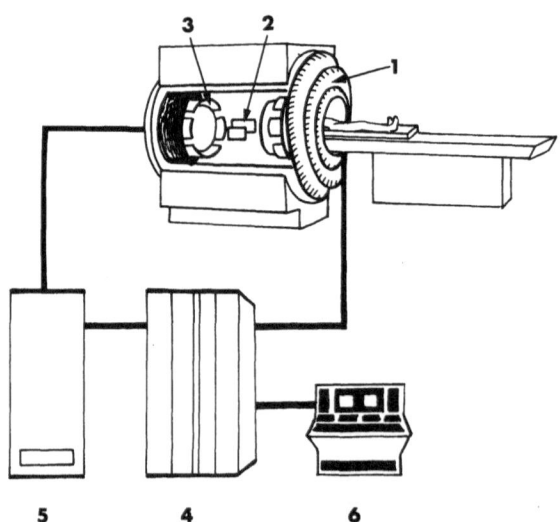

Fig. 5.2

The MR Facility

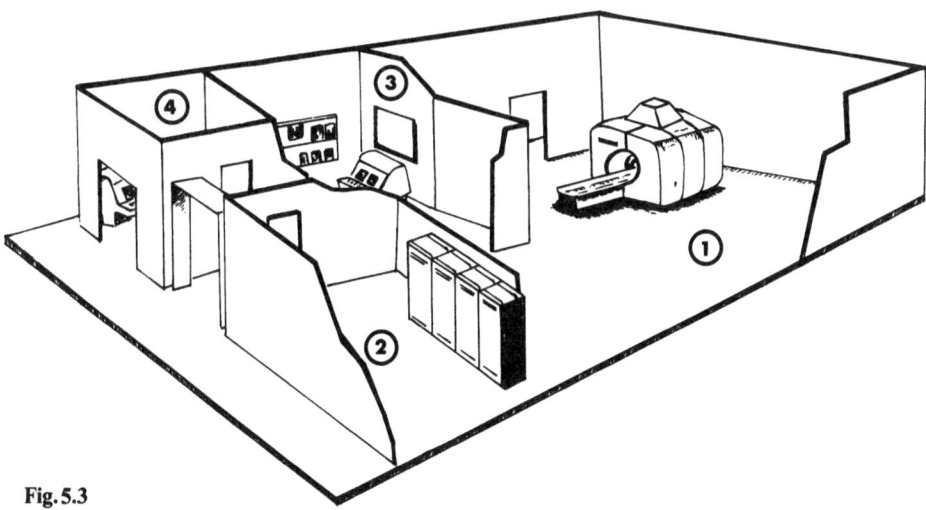

Fig. 5.3

Figure 5.3 gives a view of a MR installation:

(1) Magnet room (this has to be shielded with a Faraday cage to prevent inter-ferences between outside frequency waves and those used with the MR system).
(2) Computer room
(3) Monitoring station with console
(4) Offices (interpretation, second console, archives, etc.)

The MR Console (Fig. 5.4)

The console includes three essential elements:

(1) An image display screen
(2) One or more control monitors
(3) One or more keyboards

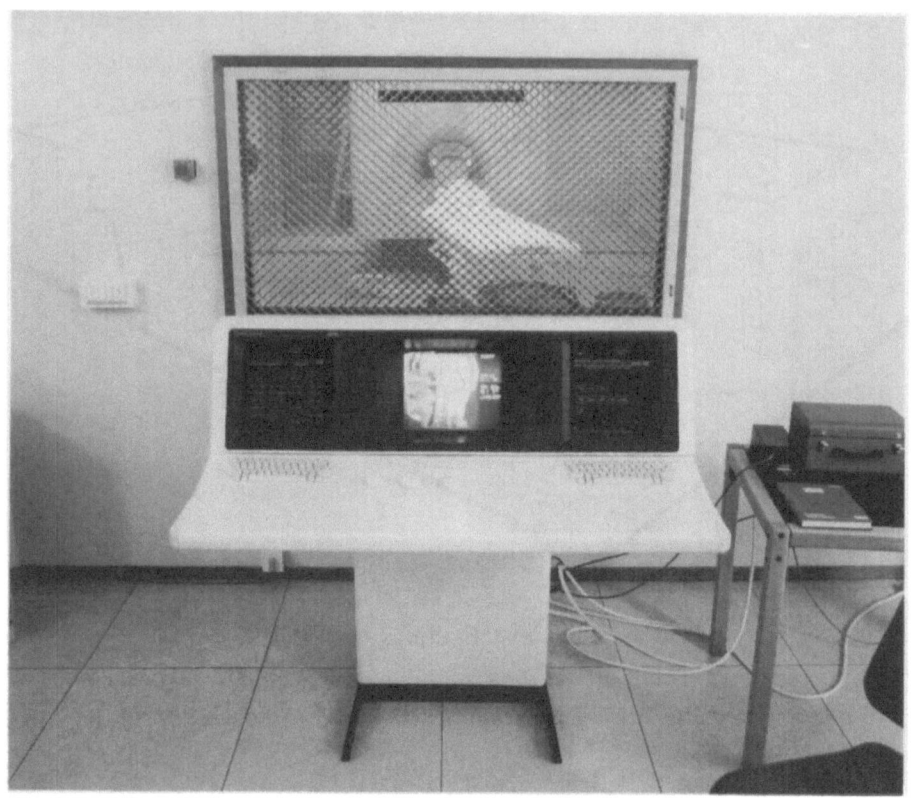

Fig. 5.4

Technical Choices

The physician performing the MR examination must reach or at least come close to a diagnosis. Two imperatives, sometimes contradictory, have to be considered:

Achieving the best possible image quality for a given sequence.
Keeping the examination time tolerable for the patient.

It is therefore important to be familiar with the effects of a range of technical decisions on image quality and examination time.

The Coil

When the protons return to equilibrium, the signal is picked up by the receiver coil. Four types of coil are currently available:

(1) Body coil (examination of thorax, abdomen and pelvis)
(2) Head coil
(3) Surface coil for visualization of relatively superficial organs (spinal cord, eye, ear, etc.) (Fig. 5.5a, $b_{1, 2}$)
(4) Local or specific organ coil with a shape adapted to that of given parts of the body (knees, elbows, hands, breasts, etc.)

The correct choice of a coil gives the best signal-to-noise ratio in the area of interest.

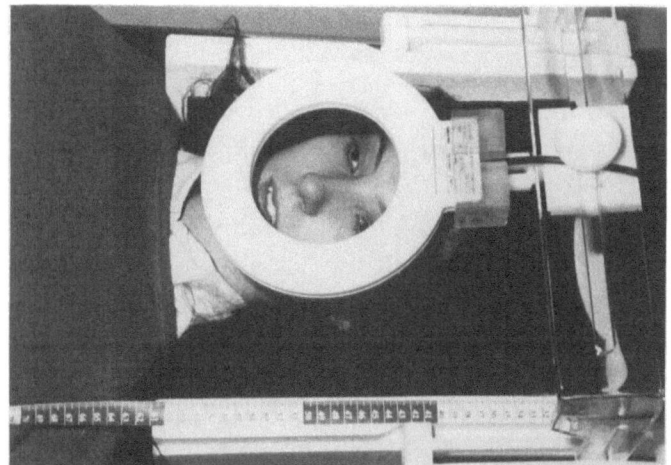

a

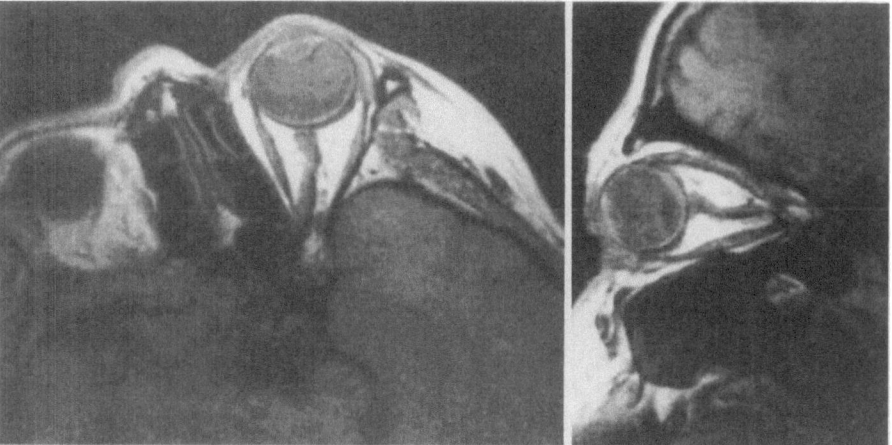

b_1 b_2

Fig. 5.5. **a** Circular surface coil. **b1, b2** Axial and sagittal sections of the left eye using a surface coil. Notice there is an almost total loss of the signal within the first few centimeters deep to the surface.

Field of View

The field of view ranges from 10 to 50 cm for most machines. Therefore, if the entire spinal cord is to be imaged in the sagittal plane, its upper and lower parts need complementary series of pulse sequences.

Slice Thickness

The basic values for slice thickness range from 3 to 15 mm (Fig.5.5c). Many machines cannot perform contiguous sections. Therefore, two successive series of images have to be made if an entire area is to be visualized.

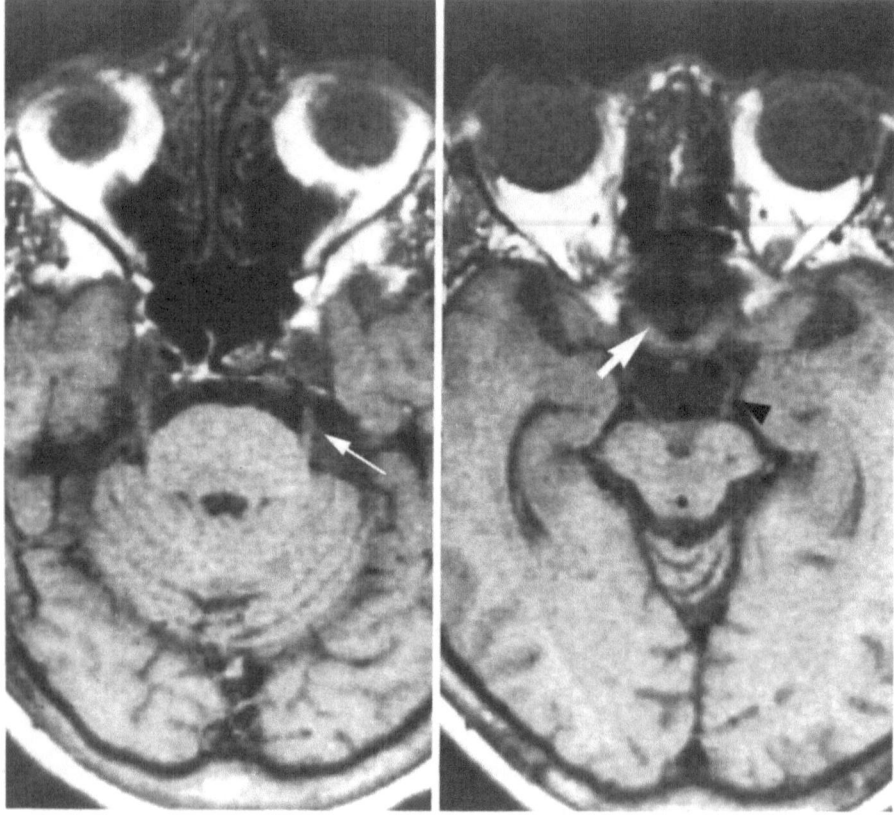

Fig.5.5c. Axial section of the brain. Slice thickness 3 mm. The optic (→), oculomotor (▶), and trigeminal (→) nerves are clearly visible

Matrix Size

In all digital imaging methods, and therefore in MR too, the image is divided up in small picture elements or *pixels*. For each individual pixel, the intensity of the MR signal is represented on a gray scale. The total of all pixels forms a *matrix* with columns and rows.

As a matter of fact, as a slice of an organ, i.e., a volume, is excited, small volume elements or *voxels* are described by analogy with pixels.

The dimensions of the matrix (i.e., the number of rows and columns) can be changed; thus, the size of voxels (and pixels) can vary. In practice, the most commonly used matrix is 256×256. Some systems offer low-resolution (128×128) and/or high-resolution (512×512) matrices.

Number of Excitations (Number of Averages)

Every individual signal needed to form a MR image can be received once or picked up several times using repeated excitations. In the latter case, the average signal value is used to generate the image. When the number of excitations is increased, the error (the noise) decreases and the measurements are more precise. In practice, the number of excitations ranges from 1 to 6 (Fig. 5.6).

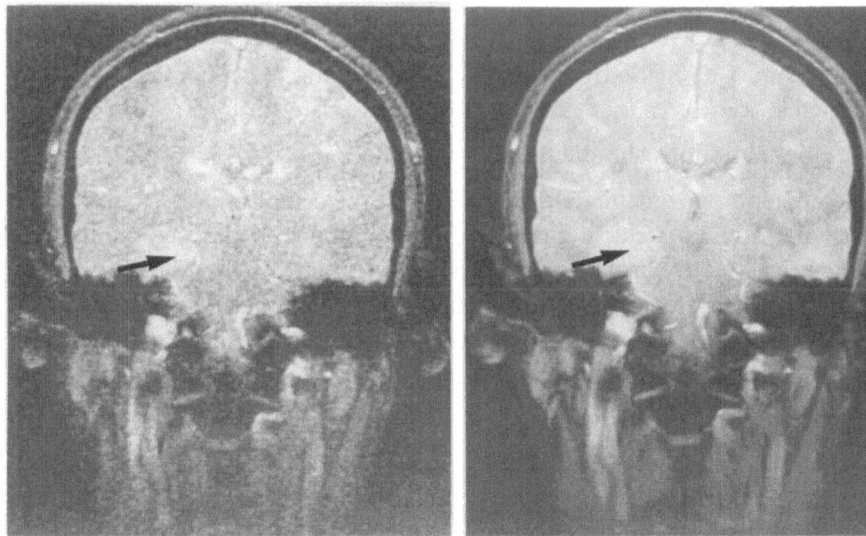

a   b

Fig. 5.6a, b. Coronal sections of the brain. Space-occupying lesion in the right temporal lobe (→). Fast imaging: TR=21 ms, TE=12 ms, $\alpha° = 30°$, matrix size 256×256. **a** One excitation; **b** Six excitations

Consequences of Technical Choices

The different choices we have just seen have implications for two major factors: image quality and image acquisition time.

Image Quality (Fig. 5.7)

The quality of an image is mainly characterized by its signal-to-noise ratio: the stronger the signal and the weaker the noise, the better the quality of the image. We must therefore strive to obtain the highest signal-to-noise ratio for each sequence. However, the quality of an image also depends on other factors, especially spatial resolution – the capacity for imaging small structures – and the signal-to-noise ratio is sometimes improved at the expense of spatial resolution.

Table 5.1 presents the possibilities for improvement of the signal-to-noise ratio and their effect on spatial resolution and acquisition time.

Table 5.1

Improvement of signal-to-noise ratio	Spatial resolution	Acquisition time	
Optimal coil		Unchanged or ↑	Unchanged
Field of view	↑	↓	Unchanged
Slice thickness	↑	↓	Unchanged
Matrix size	↓	↓	↓
Number of excitations ↑		Unchanged or ↑	↑

The choice must be made by the physician according to the pathology to be established.

Two additional notions should also be mentioned:

(1) The higher the magnetic field Bo, the better the signal-to-noise ratio (however, the optimal field, if there is one, has not yet been determined; it seems to lie between 0.5 and 1.5 Tesla). Whatever the field intensity, the quality of data processing systems plays an essential part in image quality.

(2) A long echo time (TE) and a very short repetition time (TR) lead to a decrease of the signal-to-noise ratio (see Figs. 3.7 and 3.13).

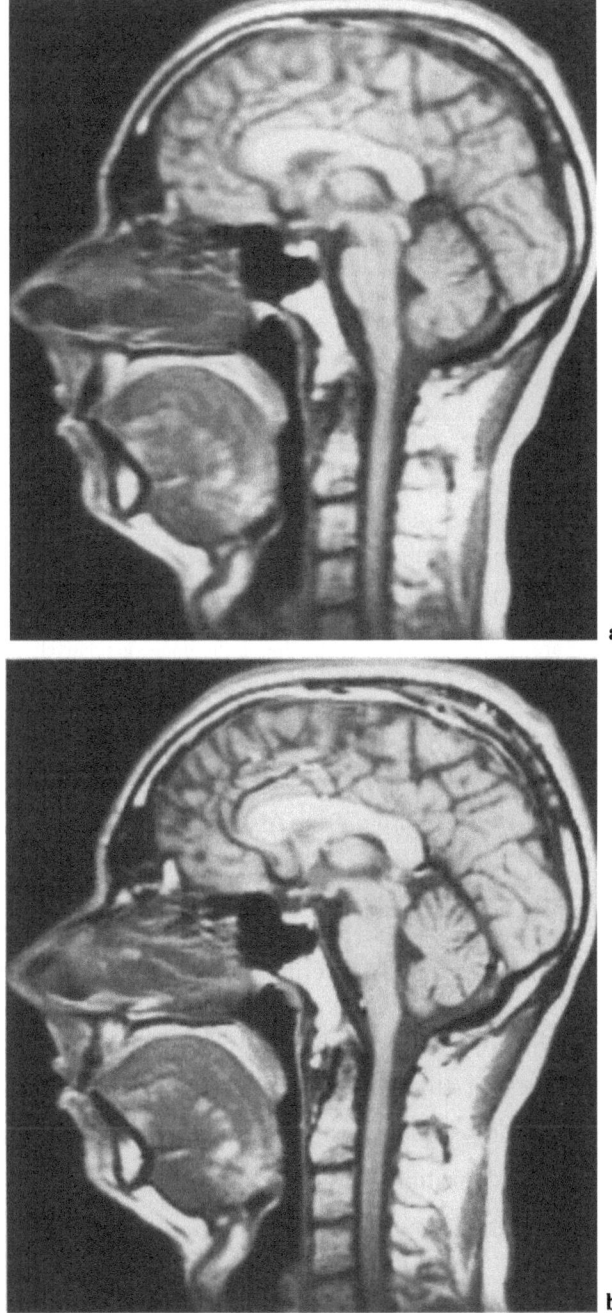

Fig. 5.7 a, b. Sagittal sections of the brain in the same patient. The pulse sequence used is the same in both cases (TR = 600 ms, TE = 20 ms). **a** Slice thickness = 10 mm, number of lines = 128, number of excitations = 1, acquisition time = 1 min and 20 s. **b** Slice thickness = 5 mm, number of lines = 256, number of excitations = 4, acquisition time = 10 min and 35 s. Note that signal-to-noise ratio and spatial resolution seem better in **b**

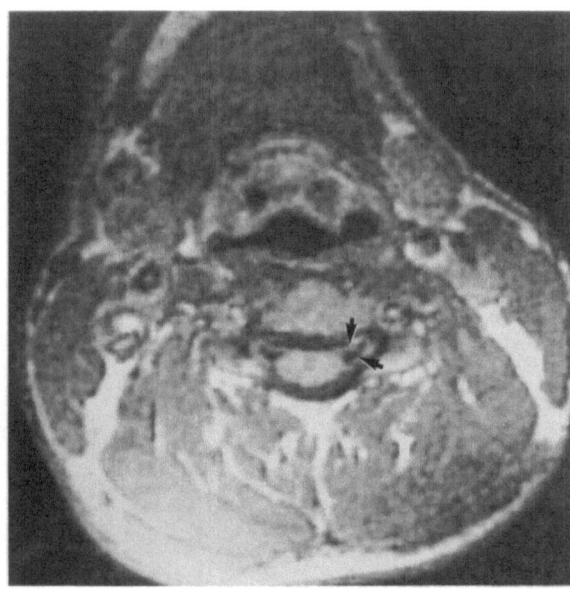

Fig. 5.8. Axial section of the cervical spine. (T1 weighting). Surface coil, slice thickness = 3 mm, matrix size = 256 × 256, four excitations. Spatial resolution is excellent, since the ventral and dorsal roots are visible (➤). On the other hand, the image is relatively noisy.

Image Acquisition Time (Examination Time)

For a given patient, the *duration* of a MR examination depends on several factors:

   Getting the patient settled and centering the area to be studied
   The number of areas to be examined
   The number and characteristics of the pulse sequences used

The examination lasts for an average of 30–90 min.

The acquisition time of a sequence is given by the following formula:

$$\text{acquisition time} = TR \times N. \times N.EX.$$

where TR is the repetition time, N. is the number of rows in the matrix, and N.EX is the number of excitations

It thus takes longer to obtain a T2-weighted sequence than a T1-weighted one, and improving the signal-to-noise ratio by increasing N.EX also increases the imaging time.

It is also easy to understand how fast imaging sequences allow for scanning 10 times shorter than in spin echo, since they use TR ranging from 20 to

200 ms. However, making up for their poor signal-to-noise ratio and achieving good image quality involves repeating the excitations 4 or 6 times or even more.

Thus a T1-weighted sequence (TR=500 ms) with two excitations and a 128-line matrix will last about 2 min, whereas a T2-weighted sequence (TR=2500 ms) with N.=256 and N.EX= 4 will last 40 min. In practice, excessively long (over 20 min) scanning times should be avoided; the longer the scanning time is, the more chance there is that the patient will move, generating artifacts that prevent the interpretation of the images (see Appendix 1).

Number of Images Obtained in One Sequence

Unlike CT, the images in MR are not acquired one at a time by the machine. All slices are generated as a whole and then displayed at the end of the sequence. The technique used is called multislice imaging and is based on the fact that a certain time elapses after the echo, which allows excitation of the neighboring slices successively (Fig. 5.9). In these conditions, the number of successive slices that can be excited in the same sequence depends principally on TR. The longer the TR, the greater the number of slices imaged.

In addition, the number of images obtained also increases with the multiple spin echo technique, since images of the 1st, 2nd, 3rd, ... nth echoes can be obtained for each slice.

Let us use again the previous example: the T1-weighted sequence produces less than 10 sections, whereas the T2-weighted one leads to 80 images (20 slices × 4 echoes for each slice).

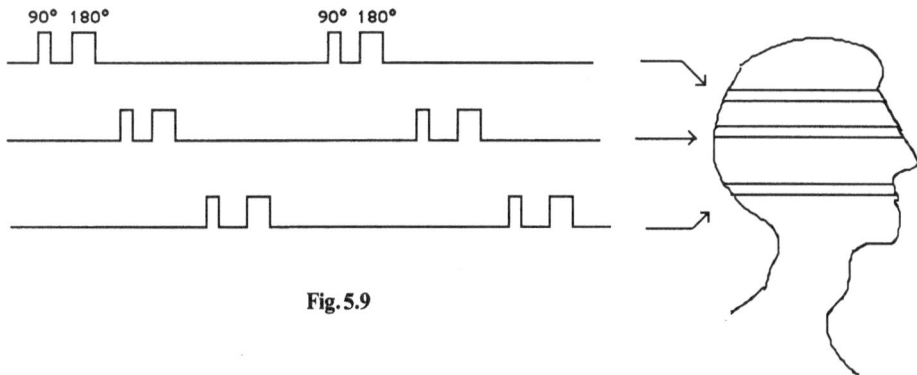

Fig. 5.9

Conclusions

Performing a MR examination demands multiple choices: first, the acquisition parameters, then the imaging plane orientation, type of coil, slice thickness, matrix size, number of excitations, etc. No definitive imaging protocols have been established as yet. However, we have provided a foundation to assist in the interpretation of MR and a practical basis for performing the examination. The following exercises using clinical cases should help the readers to check their acquisition and deficiencies.

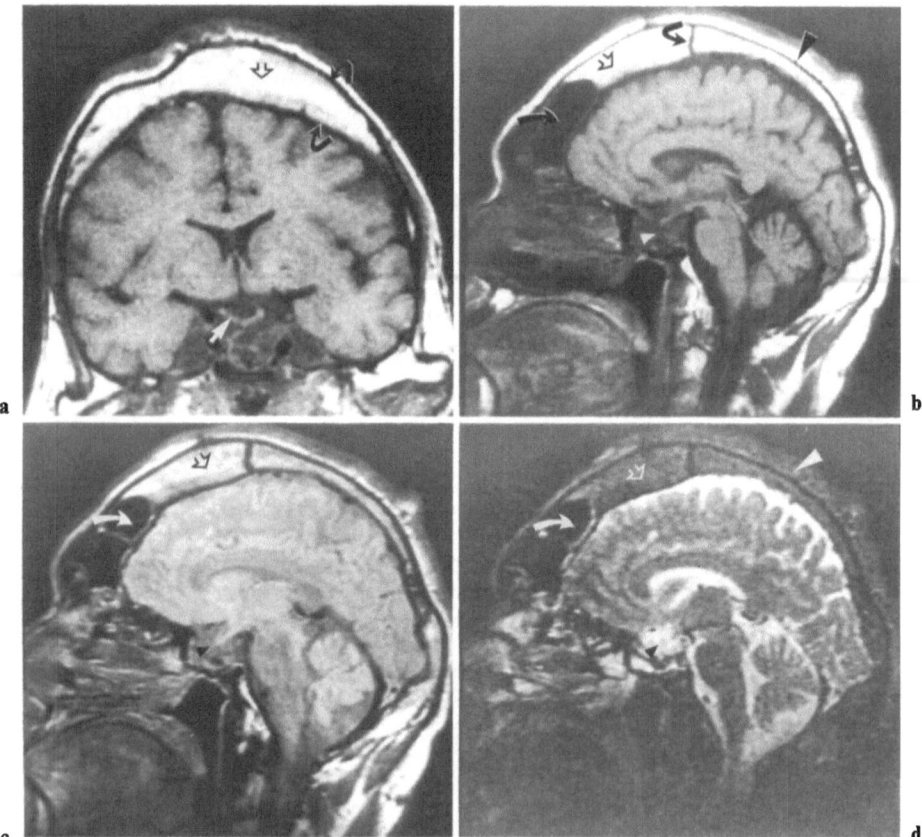

Fig. 6.1. a Frontal section across the optic chiasma. TR = 600 ms, TE = 20 ms. **b** Sagittal section. TR = 600 ms, TE = 20 ms. **c** Sagittal section. TR = 2500 ms, TE = 20 ms. **d** Sagittal section. TR = 2500 ms, TE = 100 ms

Chapter 6   **Exercises**

Exercise 1

A 47-year-old patient suffering from acromegaly and operated on for pituitary adenoma 10 years ago was referred for an abrupt decrease of visual acuity in his right eye. The examination was performed with a head coil.

Questions

(1) What is the respective T1, T2 and ρ weighting of the images in Figs. 6.1 a–d?

(2) What do you think about the morphology and signal of the cranial vault? Which element seems to be abnormal?

(3) A hypointense area can be noticed in the anterior part of the vault, on the sagittal sections ( ), whatever their weighting is. Which tissue does it correspond to?

(4) What do you find about the position of the optic chiasma (Fig. 6.1 a)? What does the signal in the pituitary sella bring to mind ( )?

(1) Figure 6.1 a, b: T1 weighting (short TR and TE); Fig. 6.1 c: mixed ρ-T1-(T2) weighting (long TR, short TE); Fig. 6.1 d: T2 weighting (long TR and TE).

(2) The vault is significantly thickened, especially in the frontal and parietal regions. This thickening affects only the diploë, a fatty structure that can be identified thanks to its hypersignal in T1 and hyposignal in T2 (⇒). Similar signals can be observed in subcutaneous fat (▶). On the other hand, the cortical substance is normal, including the sutures (↘), and gives complete hyposignal in all sequences.

(3) Such a hypointense area may correspond to cortical bone or air. In this case it is related to hyperpneumatization of the frontal sinus. The mucous membrane of the sinus is also thickened and produces a hypersignal in T2 (hyperpneumatization and mucous membrane hypertrophy are characteristic for acromegaly).

(4) There is a severe ptosis of visual pathways, especially of the optic chiasma. The signal in the pituitary fossa corresponds to a liquid structure (hypointensity in T1, hyperintensity in T2): this is the cerebrospinal fluid, which can also be found at the level of the cisterns, subarachnoid spaces and ventricles.

Conclusion. No sign of tumor recurrence, ptosis of visual pathways with empty sella turcica, frontoparietal hyperostosis, hypertrophy of the frontal sinus and of its mucous membrane.

Exercise 2

A 47-year-old patient with spinal cord astrocytoma previously treated by means of biopsy and radiotherapy. Clinical aggravation. Preoperative MRI was performed with a body coil (Fig. 6.2 a), then with a surface coil designed for examination of the spine (Figs. 6.2 b, c).

Questions

(1) On which sequence can you identify most clearly the limits of the spinal canal?

(2) Where can you set the upper and lower limits of the lesion?

(3) Can you identify one or more cystic areas in the lesion?

(4) What do you think about the area showing a hypointense signal in T2, at the upper thoracic level (Fig. 6.2a →)?

(5) What do you think about the hyperintense areas in T1 that can be seen in the vertebral bodies, especially those of C6, C7 and T1 (Fig. 6.2b →)?

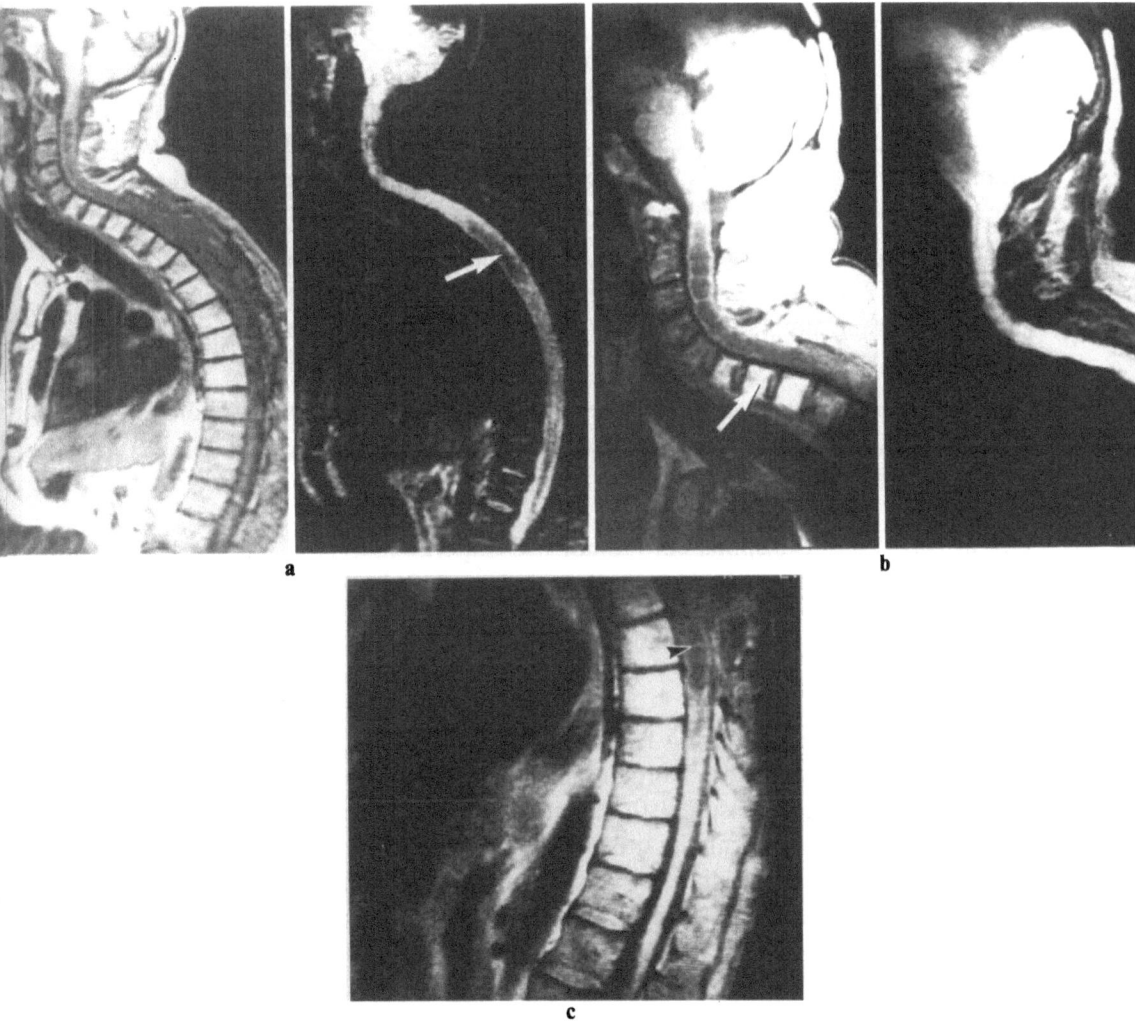

Fig. 6.2. **a** Sagittal section of the cervicodorsal spine. *Left:* TR=600 ms, TE=20 ms. *Right:* TR=2500 ms, TE=100 ms. **b** Sagittal section of the craniocervical junction and of the cervical spine. *Left* and *right:* same respective weighting as in **a**. **c** Sagittal section of the dorsolumbar spine. TR=600 ms, TE=20 ms

(1) The limits of the spinal canal appear in the T2-weighted sequence. In fact, it is not possible to differentiate the spinal cord and the subarachnoid spaces from the area of laminectomy in the T1-weighted sequence, since they all have the same hypointense signal. In the T2-weighted sequence, on the other hand, the spinal canal and its contents are clearly delineated as an area of hyperintense signal. (Therefore, the contribution of the T2-weighted sequence to diagnosis is important, even though its signal-to-noise ratio is lower than that of the T1-weighted sequence.) Note the significant dorsal kyphosis.

(2) Upper limit C1–C2; lower limit T7–T8 (the conus medullaris ends at T12–L1. The whole cord is widened from C1 to T8.

(3) Two cystic areas can be identified thanks to their hypersignal in T2: the first one extends from C2 to the upper dorsal level. The improved spatial resolution of the surface coil enables appreciation of its multi-loculated nature. The second one extends from the mid-dorsal level to T7–T8.

(4) This is the solid part of the tumor. The hypointense signal of spinal cord tumors, in T2-weighted sequences, is observed with high-field machines (1.5 Tesla); brain tumors, in contrast, often produce hyperintense signals in T2.

(5) Post-radiotherapy changes of the vertebral bodies. The hematopoietic bone marrow has been replaced by fatty tissue producing a hypersignal in T1 (and a hyposignal in T2).

Conclusion. Mid-dorsal spinal cord tumor with superior and inferior cysts. The exact nature of the tumor (astrocytoma, ependymoma or other) cannot be defined.

Exercise 3

A 28-year-old woman suffering from retrobulbar neuropathy and dizziness. Normal clinical examination. Normal paraclinical investigations, in particular evoked potentials, cerebrospinal fluid and CT. Examination was performed with a head coil. No abnormality was disclosed by the T1-weighted sequences. Notice the artifact in the right upper part of the image, mainly visible on the second echo, which is due to gradient coils misfunctioning (see Appendix 1).

Questions

(1) How would you describe the lesions?

(2) Given the morphology and MR signals, can you reach a diagnosis with certainty?

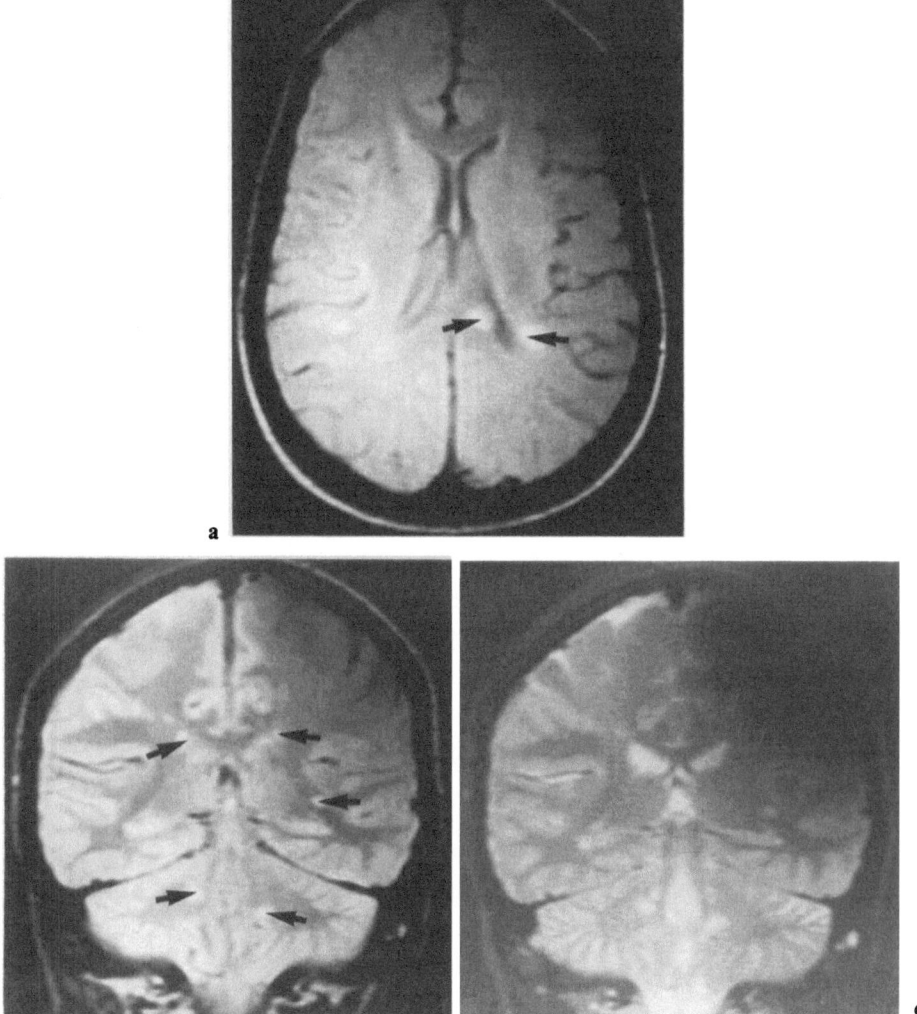

Fig. 6.3. **a** Axial section across the central part of the lateral ventricle. TR = 2000 ms, TE = 20 ms. **b** Coronal section across the cerebellum. TR = 2000 ms, TE = 40 ms. **c** Same section as in **b**. Second echo (TE = 80 ms)

71

(1) Small, round, multiple, hyperintense lesions scattered in the white matter of the cerebral and cerebellar hemispheres (→) especially the periventricular areas.

(2) No diagnosis can be made with certainty. Considering the results of the MR examination in relation to the clinical history and other investigations, the following diagnoses should be put forward (in order of probability): multiple sclerosis; sequelae of deep vascular infarcts; senile demyelination; infectious lesions. Therefore, the MR appearance of the plaques of multiple sclerosis is not specific.

Conclusion. MR aspect compatible with multiple sclerosis.

Exercise 4

A 50-year-old patient suffering from long-standing, deep epigastric pain and fever. Computerized tomography showed a heterogeneous liver with multiple hypodense masses. No primary cancer was known. The examination was performed using a body coil.

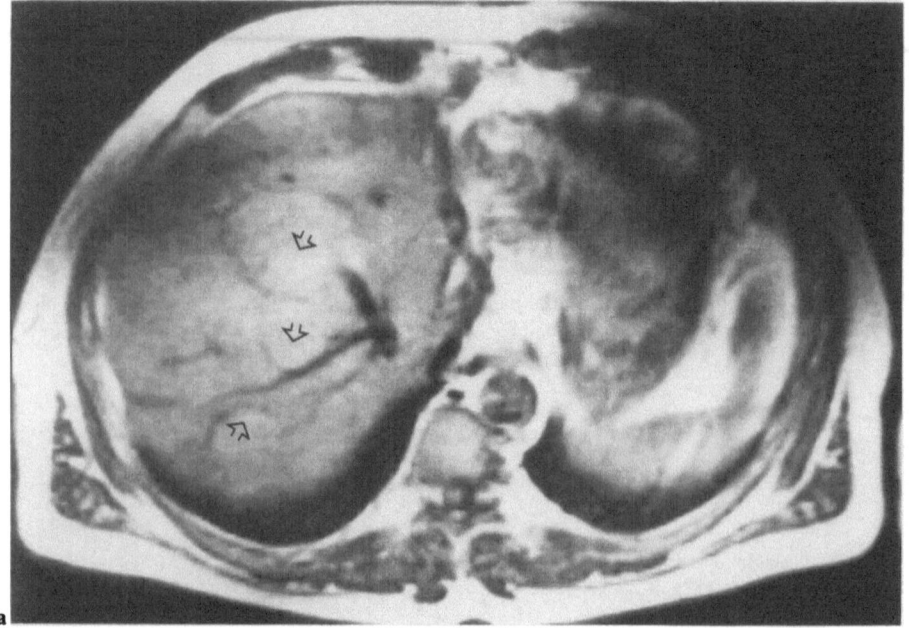

Fig. 6.4. **a** Axial section of the abdomen. TR = 800 ms, TE = 20 ms. **b** Frontal section. TR = 1500 ms, TE = 40 ms. **c** Same section as in **b**. Second echo (TE = 80 ms)

Questions

(1) Describe the location and the signals of the hepatic lesions.

(2) Which hepatic vascular structure can be seen in the coronal plane ($\rightarrow$)? Does its direction seem normal to you?

(3) Which diagnosis (or diagnoses) would you consider?

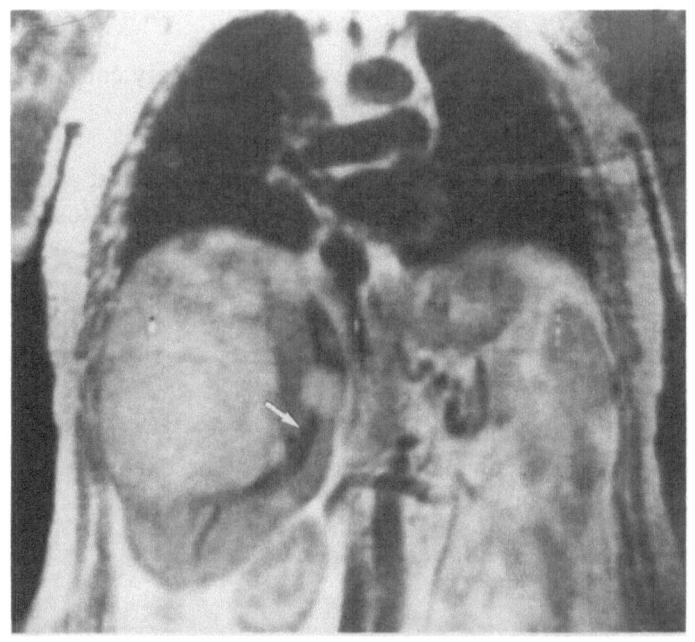

b

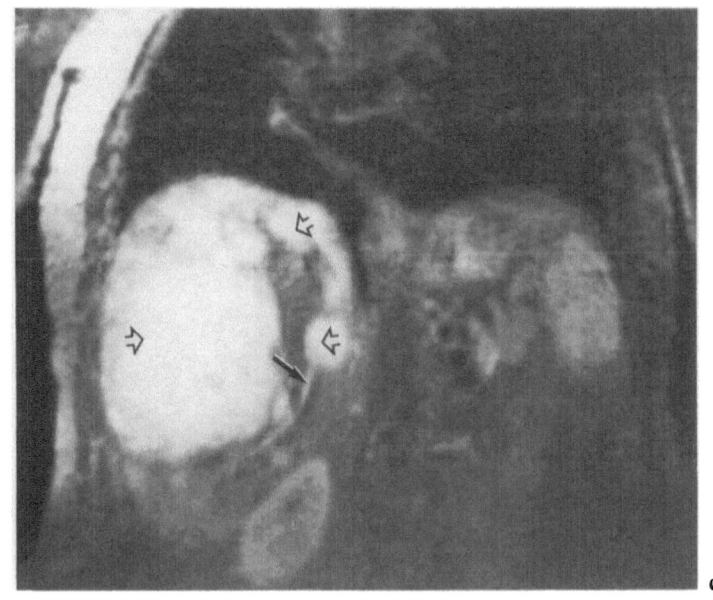

c

(1) Multiple nodular masses scattered in both hepatic lobes (⇨), with the biggest one in the right lobe. These lesions are relatively homogeneous and show a hyperintense signal when compared with the adjacent normal parenchyma, especially in the T2-weighted sequence.

(2) This is the right portal vein displaced inferiorly and to the left by the biggest nodule.

(3) No certain diagnosis can be put forward. The primary considerations are multinodular hepatoma or multiple metastases.

Conclusion. Diffuse, multinodular masses, scattered in the liver and displacing the right portal vein inferiorly. Multinodular hepatoma or diffuse metastases are most likely.

Exercise 5

A 6-year-old child with bilateral pes cavus and moderate sphincter dysfunction. L5–S1 spina bifida on plain radiographs. The examination was performed with a surface coil.

Questions

(1) What is the spinal cord anomaly?

(2) There is a lesion behind the terminal part of the spinal cord (→). Can you characterize it? Can you determine its extension?

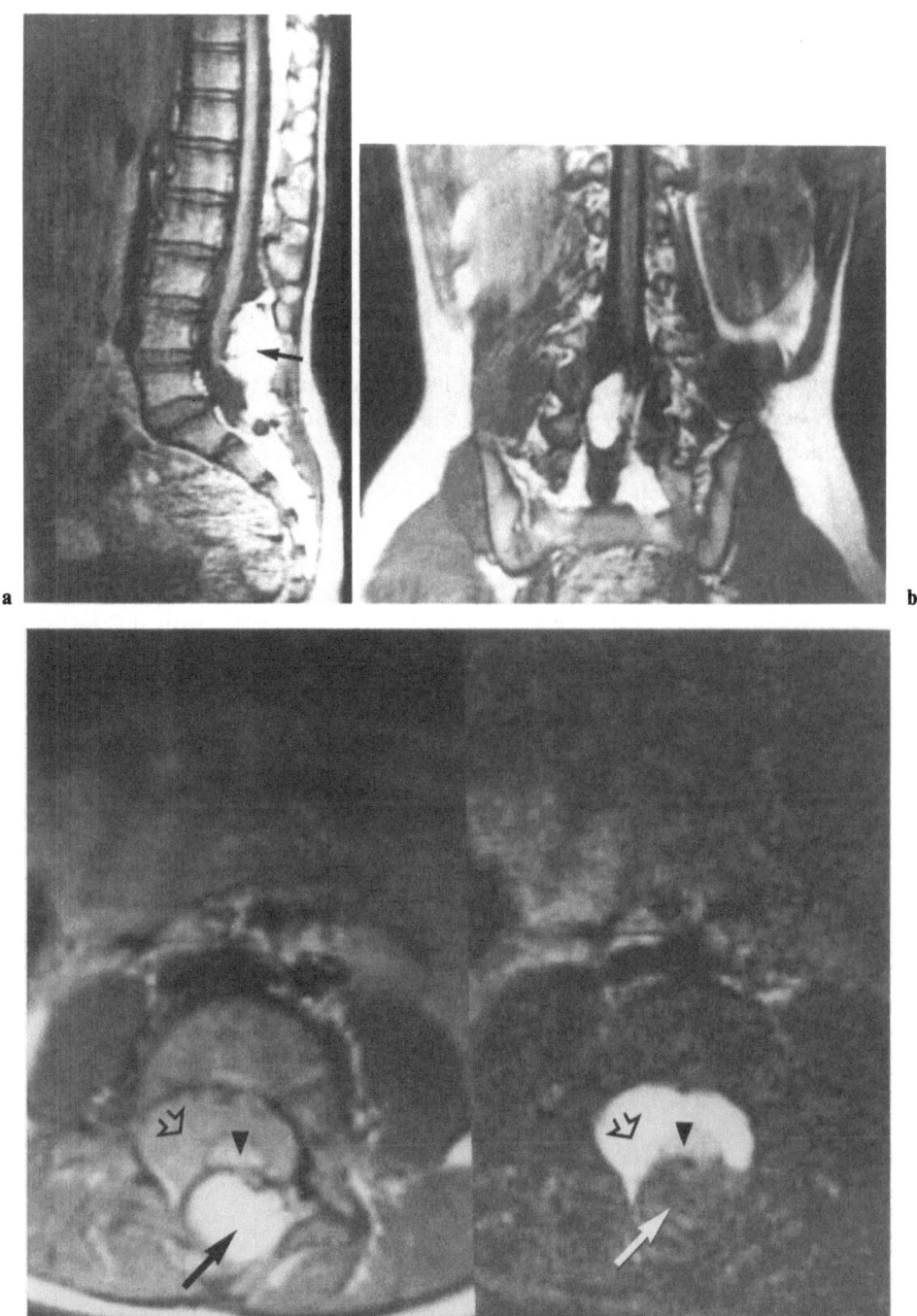

Fig. 6.5. **a** Sagittal section of the lumbosacral spine. TR = 600 ms, TE = 20 ms. **b** Frontal section. Same weighting as in Fig. **a**. **c** Axial section across L4. TR = 2000 ms. *Left:* first echo, TE = 25 ms; *right:* fourth echo, TE = 100 ms (images of second and third echoes not shown)

(1) Tethered cord ending at the level of L5. The cord does not show any abnormal signal.

(2) The mass in contact with the cord produces a hypersignal in T1 and a hyposignal in T2 that are characteristic for fatty tissue: it is a lipoma extending from L4–L5 into the sacral canal. On the axial sections, the relationship between the spinal cord (▶), the lipoma (➔) and the cerebrospinal fluid (⇨) are clearly depicted. (Notice in particular the enlargement of the spinal canal).

Conclusion. Tethered cord ending at L5, large lumbosacral lipoma.
MR has become a primary modality in the preoperative assessment of spinal dysraphism.

Exercise 6

A 50-year-old patient suffering from recent left hemiparesis with headache. Angiography shows a large arteriovenous malformation (Fig. 6.6 a). MR examination was performed with a head coil (Fig. 6 b, c). The images 6.6 d and e were taken 3 days after embolization of the malformation.

Questions

(1) Can you identify the venous sac?

(2) What effects does the malformation have on the cerebral parenchyma?

(3) What changes can you observe in the venous sac when you compare its appearance before and after embolization?

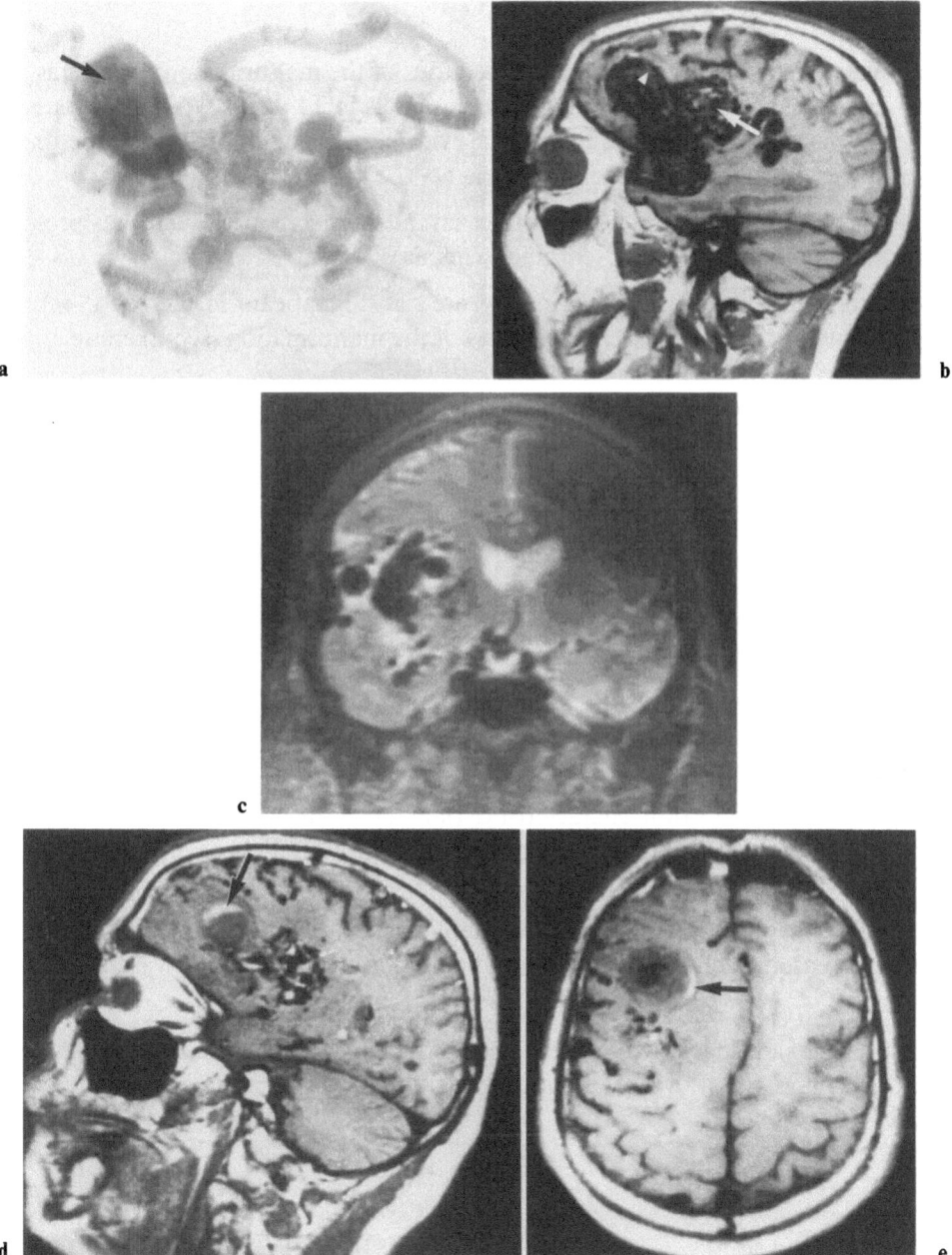

Fig. 6.6. **a** Right carotid angiography (lateral view). The ectatic venous sac (→) is located anterior to the nidus of the arteriovenous malformation. **b** Right parasagittal section of the brain. TR = 600 ms, TE = 25 ms. **c** Coronal section. TR = 2500 ms, TE = 90 ms. **d** Right parasagittal section performed 3 days after embolization. TR = 600 ms, TE = 25 ms. **e** Axial section across the upper part of the malformation. Examination performed 3 days after embolization. TR = 600 ms, TE = 25 ms

Answers

(1) Yes, thanks to arteriography ... The nidus of the malformation appears as an area of punctate hypersignals and hyposignals in T1 and T2 (→), whereas the venous sac has a global hyposignal with curvilinear hypersignals due to turbulence phenomena inside the ectasia (▶).

(2) The malformation has a mass effect on the lateral ventricles and has produced atrophy of the insula (chronic ischemia).

(3) After embolization, a hyperintense area in T1 appears in the sac (→), thus showing the progressive thrombosis of the malformation (see Exercise 7).

Conclusion. Large right frontoparietal arteriovenous malformation before and after embolization.

Flow Effects in MRI (Fig. 6.7)

Flowing fluids (mainly blood, but also cerebrospinal fluid) present peculiar and complex problems for MR, as the case we have seen demonstrates.

In routine pulse sequences (i.e., spin echo), the vessels are often spontaneously visible. Their signal (hyperintense, hypointense or even mixed) depends on three main factors:

Flow velocity and flow characteristics (laminar or turbulent)
Position of the vessel relative to the section plane (parallel or perpendicular)
Acquisition parameters (TR, TE, etc.).

With fast imaging, flowing fluids are often imaged with a hyperintense signal; for that reason, such sequences should be used in the detection of vascular lesions.

Lastly, there are special sequences aimed at making vascular structures visible and at quantifying flows. These sequences do not yet form a part of routine MR.

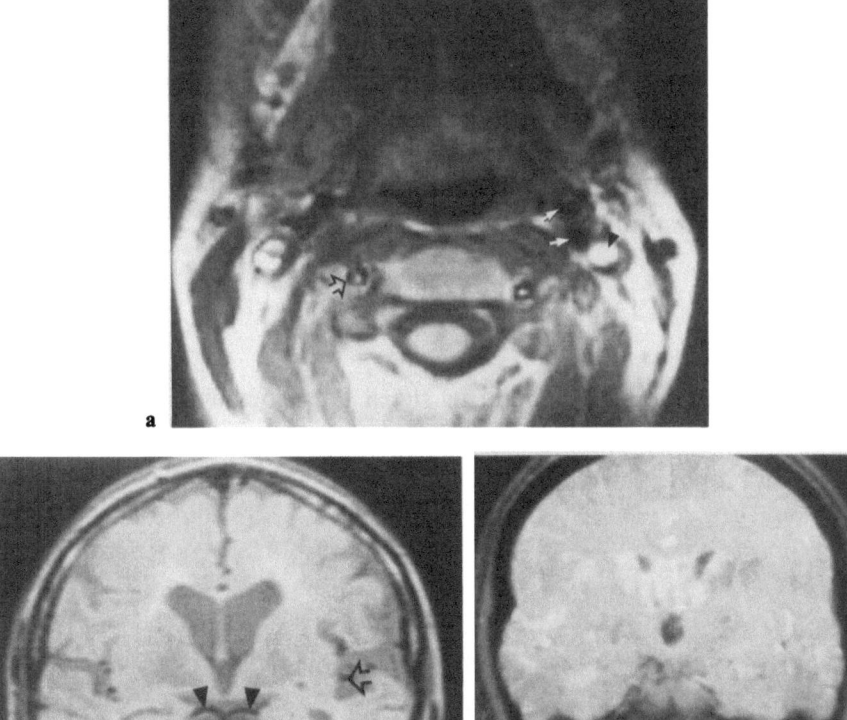

Fig. 6.7. **a** Axial section across C3. TR = 500 ms, TE = 20 ms. It is possible to identify the vertebral arteries in the foramen transversarium (⇗; central hyperintensity, peripheral hypointensity), the internal jugular vein (▶), and the carotid arteries (→). Note on the *left,* that the internal jugular vein appears as a hyperintense structure and the internal and external carotids as hypointense structures. **b** Frontal section of the brain at the level of the pontine cisterns. Spin echo: TR = 2000 ms, TE = 20 ms. The basilar artery (↘), the vertebral arteries (→), and the posterior cerebral arteries (▶) appear as hypointense structures; the Sylvian arteries and some of their collaterals (⇗) can also be identified. **c** Coronal section. Fast imaging: TR = 21 ms, TE = 12 ms, α° = 30°. The vertebral arteries are visualized all along their cervical course (→). The internal jugular veins are also shown with a hyperintense signal (⇗)

Exercise 7

Twenty-year-old patient with previous history of headache. Abrupt cerebellar syndrome. The initial CT (Fig. 6.8 a) showed a pontine mass with a hypodense center and a hyperdense periphery that does not enhance with contrast media (→). Arteriography was normal. The admitted diagnosis was tumor of the brain stem. Radiotherapy was started. The MR examination, requested 1 month later to confirm the diagnosis, was performed using a head coil.

Questions

(1) Describe the lesion, its site and its signal intensities in the different sequences.

(2) Can you propose a diagnosis?

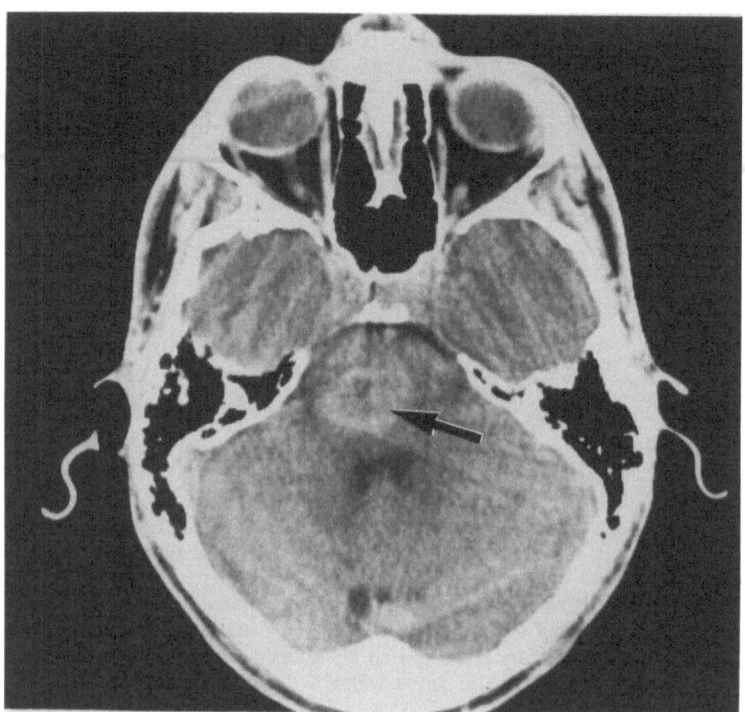

Fig. 6.8 a. Initial CT.

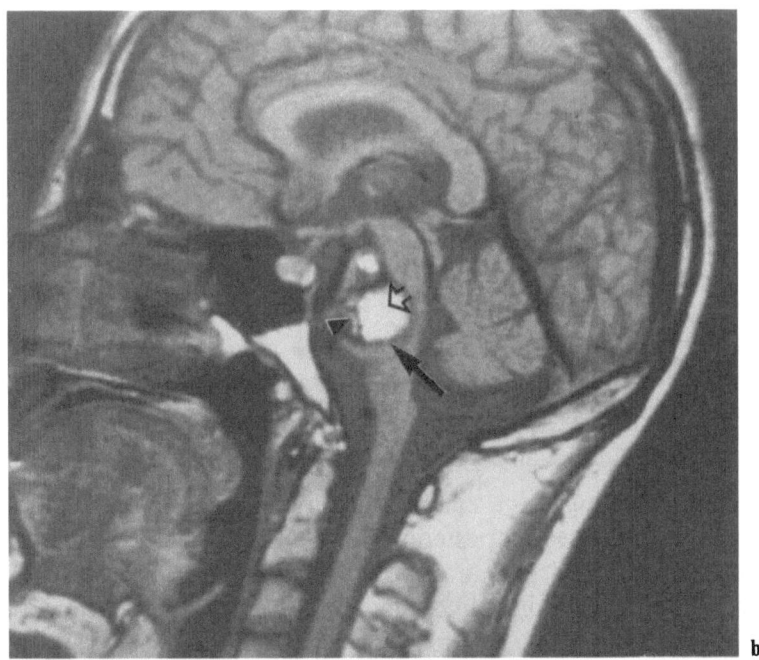

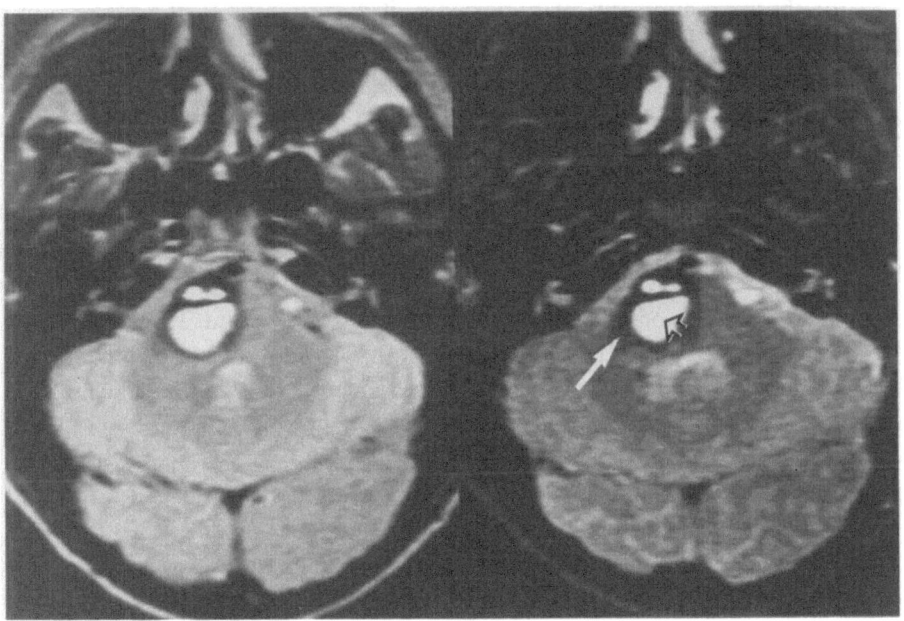

Fig. 6.8 b, c. **b** Median sagittal section. TR = 600 ms, TE = 20 ms. **c** Axial section at the level of the facial and vestibulocochlear nerves. TR = 2000 ms. *Left:* first echo (TE = 50 ms); *right:* second echo (TE = 100 ms).

(1) Location: space-occupying lesion located in the pons, slightly lateralized to the right, deforming the contour of the brain stem on the right, producing no mass effect on the fourth ventricle.

Signals:

The anterior part shows mixed hyperintense and hypointense signals in the T1-weighted image (▶) and a hyperintense signal in the T2-weighted ones.

The posterior and largest part of the lesion appears as a hypersignal in T1 and T2 (⇨).

The whole lesion is surrounded by a peripheral rim of marked hyposignal, particularly visible in the T2-weighted imaged (➔).

(2) The lesion should be analyzed as follows:

The anterior part suggests a small vascular malformation (see Exercise 6).

The hypersignal observed posteriorly in T1 and T2 corresponds to a subacute hematoma. The degradation products of hemoglobin (especially methemoglobin) account for these hypersignals (paramagnetic behavior, see Exercise 8).

As for the peripheral rim of hyposignal, it corresponds to the resorption granuloma of the hematoma. This granuloma contains macrophages filled with hemosiderin (final by-product of hemoglobin). The ferric atoms of hemosiderin are modifying the magnetic field Bo, thus creating a kind of "magnetic black hole" where excitation of the protons can no longer be performed.

A second MRI examination was performed 5 months later (Fig. 6.8 d, e). Neurological assessment had returned to normal values.

How has the lesion evolved?

A marked decrease of the posterior hypersignal in T1 and T2 can be observed (progressive lysis of the clot). On the other hand, the area of mixed hyper- and hyposignals is still observed (persistence of the vascular malformation).

Conclusion. Occult vascular malformation of the brain stem (normal arteriography) with subacute hemorrhage.
Radiotherapy was interrupted after the first MR examination.

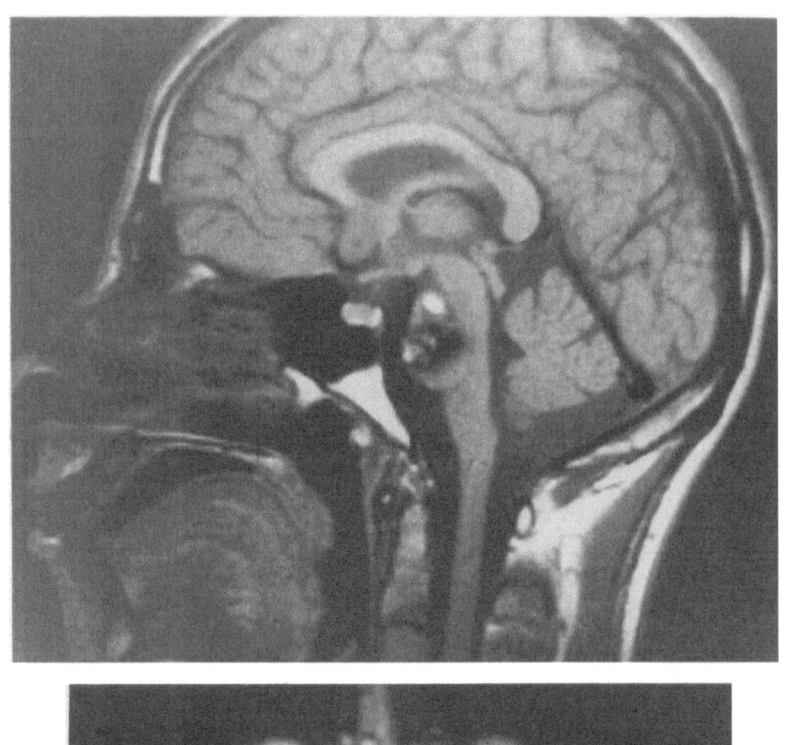

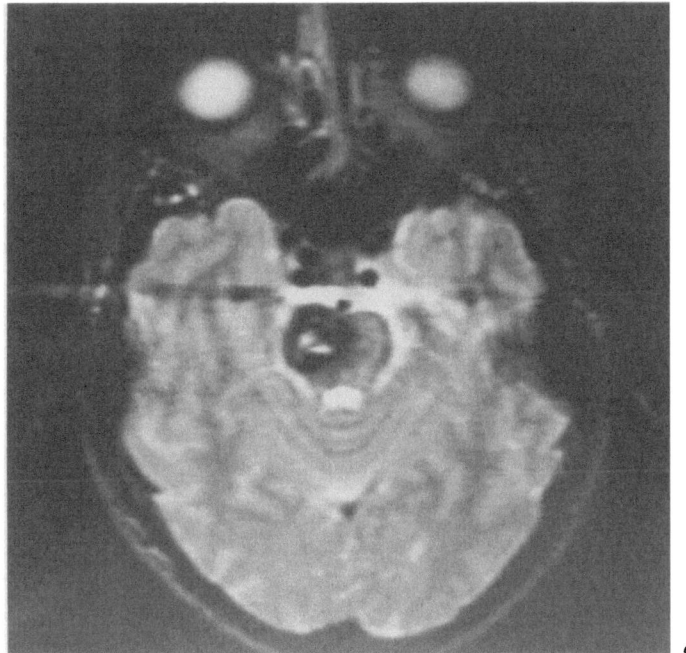

Fig. 6.8 d, e. d Sagittal section. Same parameters as for **b**. Examination performed 6 months after clinical onset. **e** Axial section (plane of imaging has a different obliquity from that of **c**). TR = 2000 ms, TE = 100 ms. Examination performed 6 months after clinical onset

Exercise 8

53-year-old female suffering from long-standing, resistant headaches. Normal neurological assessment. CT (Fig. 6.9 a, b) showed a partially calcified, hyperdense, right paracavernous lesion, enhancing with contrast and suggesting a calcified aneurysm of the carotid. However, angiography was normal. Two diagnoses were therefore evoked: thrombosed carotid aneurysm and tumor. MR examination was performed using a head coil.

Questions

(1) What morphological abnormalities and abnormal signal intensities can be observed in Fig. 6.9 c, d?

(2) How do you account for the area of hypersignal in the right paracavernous region seen in Fig. 6.9 e, f?

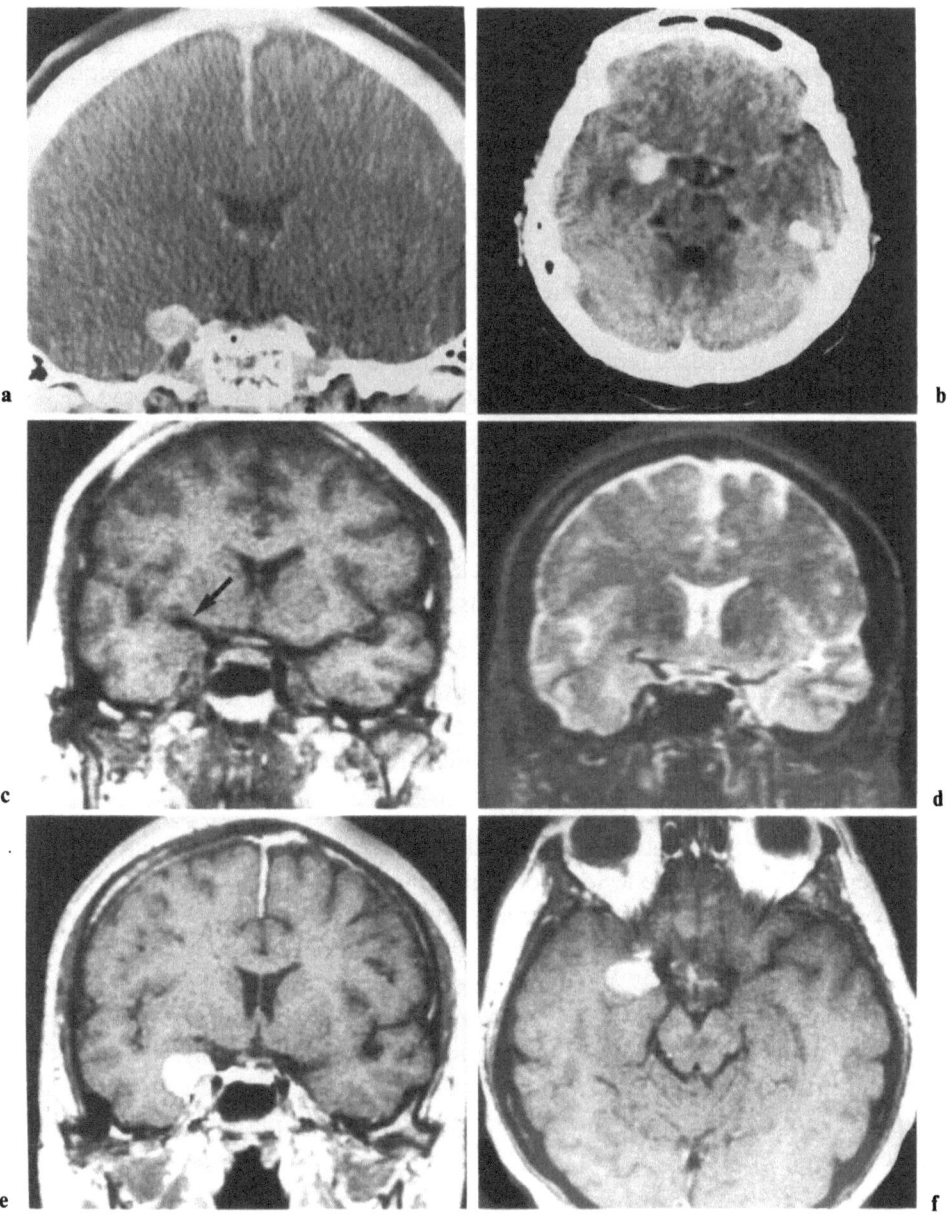

Fig. 6.9. **a** Non-contrast CT (coronal plane). **b** Contrast CT (axial plane). **c** Coronal section across the cavernous sinuses. TR = 600 ms, TE = 20 ms. **d** Same imaging plane as for **c**. TR = 3000 ms, TE = 100 ms. **e** Same imaging plane and same parameters as for **c**. **f** Axial section. Same parameters as for **c**

(1) No signal abnormality in T1- and T2-weighted sequences; in particular, no hypersignals indicating vascular thrombosis (see Exercise 7). The first part of the right middle cerebral artery is slightly elevated (mass effect; →).

(2) The acquisition parameters (TR, TE, matrix dimensions, slice thickness, etc.) have not changed. The hypersignal is caused by injection of gadolinium-DTPA (Schering, Laboratories). Note that the lower part of the mass is in contact with the base of the skull, therefore with the meninges.

Conclusion. Dural-based, enhancing, right paracavernous mass. The most likely diagnosis is meningioma (this diagnosis was confirmed by pathology).

Paramagnetic Substances. Contrast Media in MRI

Paramagnetic substances shorten the relaxation times of the tissue in which they are injected (therefore a hyperintense signal can be observed in T1 and a hypointense signal in T2).

Some paramagnetic substances are by-products of pathological alterations. The best-studied substances are the degradation products of hemoglobin (deoxyhemoglobin and methemoglobin) which are found in hematomas (see Exercise 7).

On the other hand, contrast media with paramagnetic properties have been developed. They enhance lesions (or parts of lesions) which have a poor natural contrast with the surrounding tissue, thus making them clearly visible.
The substance used for examination of the human body is gadolinium combined with DTPA (or DOTA) administered by means of intravenous injection. The pharmacodynamic properties of these products are similar to those of the contrast media used in conventional radiology; more specifically, it results in enhancement of vascularized tumors and penetrates a disrupted blood-brain barrier. No serious adverse effects (allergic reactions, in particular) have been observed, as yet.

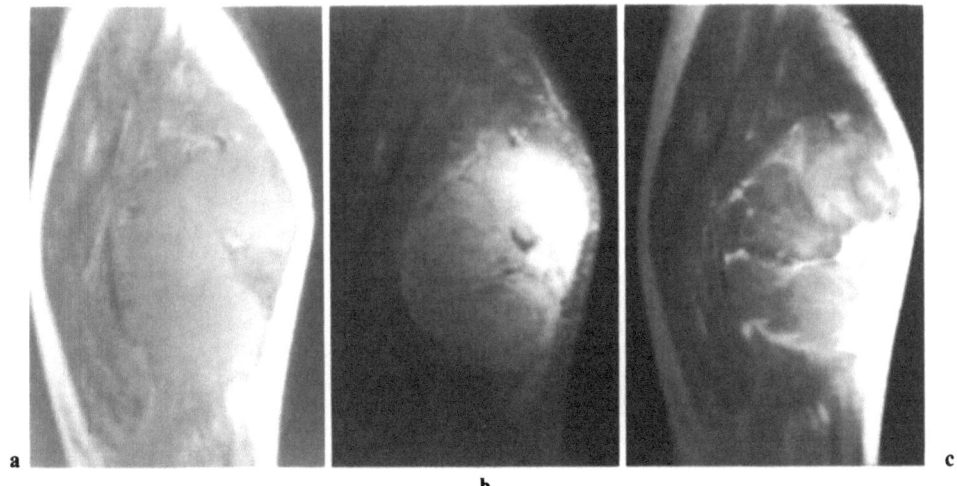

a   c

b

Fig. 6.10a–c. Undifferentiated sarcoma of the calf. Sagittal sections. **a** T1-weighted sequence.
b T2-weighted sequence. **c** T1-weighted sequence. Injection of gadolinium-DTPA. The vascularized parts of the tumor take up the contrast medium and appear as hyperintense structures

Appendix

1. Artifacts

It is necessary to be familiar with the specific artifacts appearing in MR, since they can conceal pathological elements or simulate pathology that does not exist. The list of different artifacts gets longer every day, but we shall mention only the ones most frequently recorded.

Motion Artifacts

Motion artifacts may appear because the patient has moved (trembling, inadequate immobilization, etc.) and have a characteristic appearence in the direction of the motion. Since all images in one sequence are taken at the same time (see p. 65), it is important not to use excessively long sequences, for one movement spoils all images.

Cardiac and respiratory motions often give rise to artifacts concealing the surrounding organs. However, they can be reduced by cardiac and/or respiratory gating and by resorting to fast imaging (the patient does not breathe during the 5–15 s each "minisequence" lasts). Synchronization with EKG is also used to visualize cardiac structures at different stages of the cardiac cycle.

Lastly, blood and to a lesser extent cerebrospinal fluid give rise to various artifacts that can be divided into two categories. The first category comprises those artifacts which are "predictable" for those already acquainted with flow phenomena in MR. Detailed explanation would be too far beyond the scope of this book. The second category includes artifacts similar to cardiac and respiratory ones. These create "ghost" images lying outside blood vessels and subarachnoid spaces and may sometimes pose serious problems of interpretation.

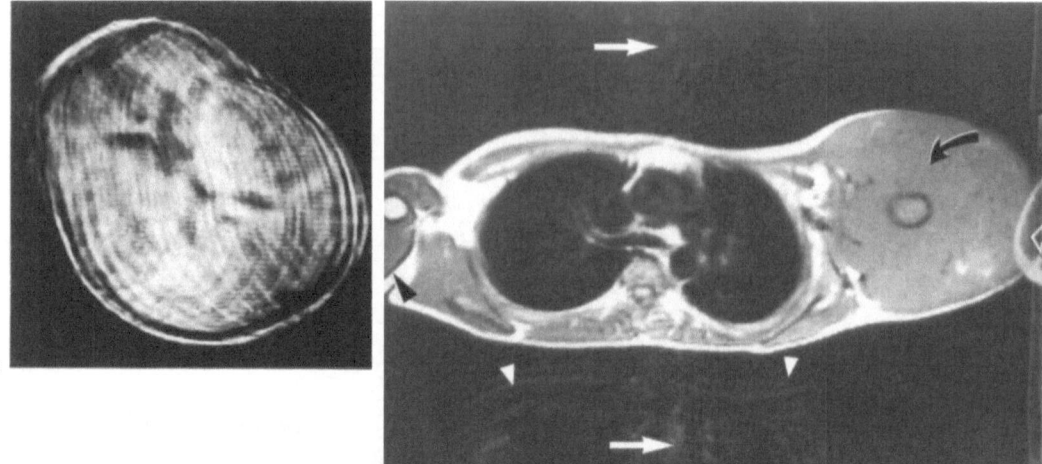

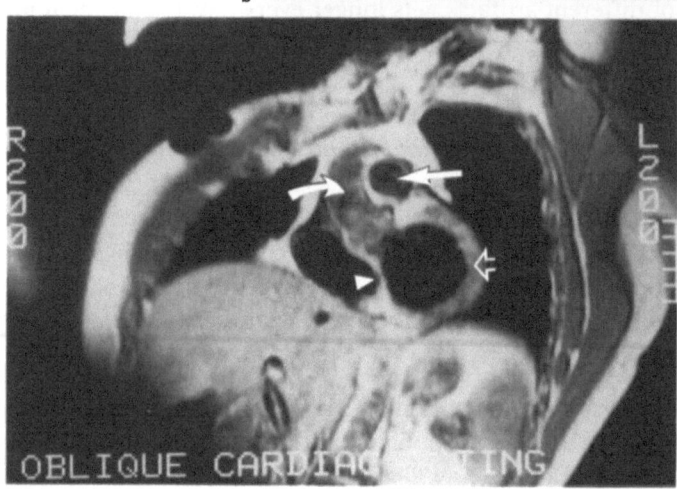

Fig. A.1.1 a–c. **a** Axial section of the brain. Major artifacts caused by motion of the head. **b** Axial section through the superior part of the thorax. Left humeral osteosarcoma (⌇). Four artifacts can be seen on this image: respiratory motion artifacts, reproducing the chest wall (▶); flow artifact (→); "wrap-around" of the right arm into the left side of the image (▶); chemical shift artifact (⟡). **c** Oblique section of the thorax through the cardiac chambers. Sequence synchronized with EKG. It is possible to identify the left ventricular wall (⟡), the interventricular septum (▶), the ascending aorta (⌇) and the main pulmonary artery (→).

Fig. A.1.1 d–g. **d** Axial section of the thorax performed without cardiac gating. The main cardiac structures cannot be identified. Notice the extent of motion artifacts projecting in front of and behind the mediastinum. **e** Thoracoabdominal frontal section. Right adrenal adenoma (→). Fast imaging, with the patient holding his breath during data acquisition (acquisition time: 11 s). There are no respiratory motion artifacts, but cardiac artifacts are still visible (⟡). A chemical shift artifact can also be noticed, surrounding the kidneys (⌇). **f** Sagittal section of the brain. Artifact from dental bridgework (→). The artifact is relatively limited and does not prevent analysis of intracranial structures. **g** Artifact from hairpin, with the typical pattern: central signal dropout, peripheral hyperintense rim, distortion of the surrounding anatomic structures

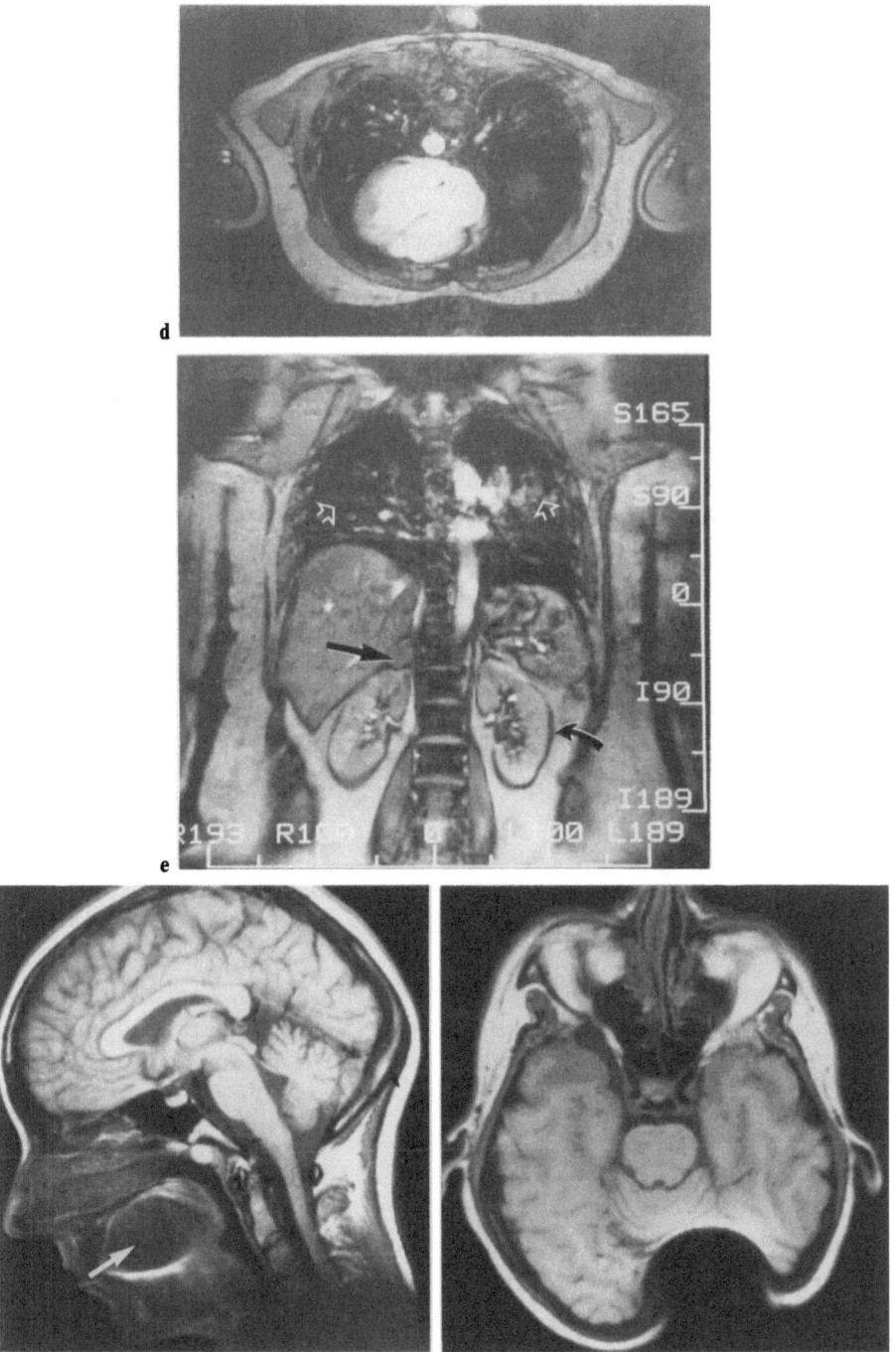

Metal Objects

Ferromagnetic objects (dental prostheses, orthopedic prostheses, etc.) produce characteristic artifacts in the form of a central hypointense signal area surrounded by a peripheral area of hypersignal, and of distortion of the neighboring structures.

Nonferromagnetic implants (hip prostheses, etc.) can produce similar but less marked artifacts.

Chemical Shift Artifacts

Chemical shift artifacts appear at the interfaces between water and fat because the precessional frequency of protons is slightly different in these two substances. This leads to misregistration of the signals when they are displayed by the machine: the interfaces overlap (hyperintense signal) or part (hypointense signal).

Wrap-Around/Aliasing

Wrap-around or aliasing appears when the diameter of the scanned area is greater than the dimensions of the field of view used: a part of the image is "folded" on itself.

System Malfunction

Malfunction of the MRI apparatus may take any one of several forms: inhomogeneity of the magnetic field B_o, improper adjustment of radiofrequency pulses, malfunction of coils (transmitter/receiver coil, gradient coils), etc.

2. Signal Localization

We know that each kind of tissue has given values for ρ, T1 and T2. Therefore, the MR signal varies from one tissue to another. Yet imaging involves being able to analyze the contribution to ρ, T1 and T2 of every point (voxel) of the image; i.e., determining the position of each organ in the final image.

This is a technical problem, which is not necessary to understand in order to interpret MR images. We have nevertheless chosen to give a (brief) explanation of signal location here because it allows for more precise study of some images, especially when flows and artifacts have to be taken into account.

Slice Selection

We have seen that excitation involves providing the protons with a given amount of energy (exactly equal to the difference between the energy levels of excited and non-excited protons, see note 2, p. 9). Energy, and more specifically the frequency ω (omega) of the energy-carrying wave, depend on the intensity of the magnetic field Bo, according to the Larmor equation:

$$\omega = \gamma \cdot Bo$$

The "gyromagnetic ratio" γ (gamma) is constant for a specific type of nucleus: for instance, $\gamma = 42.58$ Mhz/Tesla for the hydrogen nucleus.

Since radiofrequency waves are not focused in MRI, and thus spread in all directions, a given imaging plane can be selected according to the following principle: the intensity of Bo is modified everywhere, except in the area where protons are to be excited. To achieve this result, a linear and oriented variation is superimposed over Bo, i.e., a *magnetic field gradient* (generated using gradient coils). Thus the ω-frequency wave will excite only the protons located in the area where the magnetic field has the exact intensity of Bo. No excitation occurs, and of course no MR signal is generated, in the areas where field intensity is Bo $\pm \Delta$b, i.e., weaker or stronger than Bo.

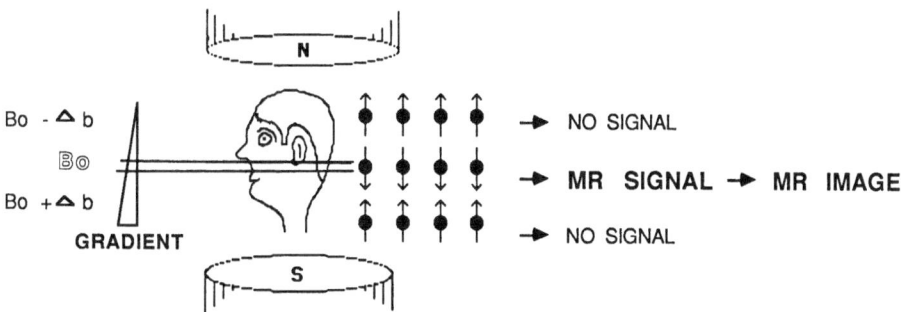

Fig. A.2.1

Differentiating Protons in One Slice (Fig. A.2.2)

Once the section plane has been selected (Fig. A.2.2a), the signals coming from each point of the slice have to be differentiated. In this case, too, magnetic field gradients are used.

The first gradient is applied in one direction of the slice (for instance, the X direction in Fig. A.2.2b): in the direction of the gradient, and because of its action, protons precess at slightly different speeds (according to the intensity of the gradient) and thus have different phase angles which make it possible to differentiate them. This operation is called *phase encoding*.

A second gradient (called "read-out gradient") is applied in a direction perpendicular to that of the first gradient (Fig. A.2.2c): it gives rise to phase angle differences in each band of protons which previously had the same phase angle. In this case, too, the new proton phase angles provide spatial information. This operation is called *frequency encoding*.

The method we have described (the most commonly used) is called "2DFT" (two-dimensional Fourier transform).

Lastly, we have seen that in fast imaging, echoes may be produced using "gradient reversal" (see p.33). A read-out gradient is applied very briefly, causing dephasing of the protons. The gradient is then immediately reversed, causing rephasing of the protons: an echo is then produced.

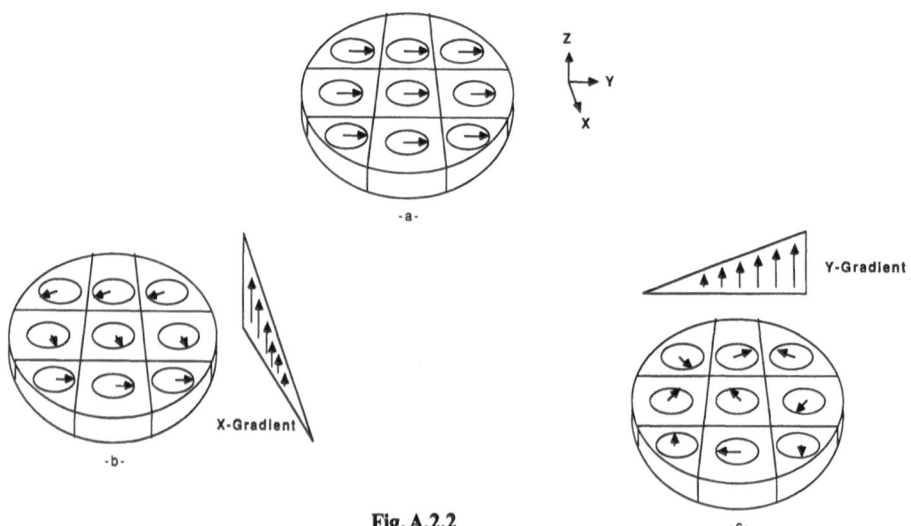

-a-

X-Gradient

-b-

Y-Gradient

-c-

Fig. A.2.2

94

Selected Bibliography

Physics, Tissue Parameters, Pulse Sequences

American College of Radiology Glossary of MR terms (1986). American College of Radiology, Reston, Va

Bradley WG, Newton TH, Crooks LE (1983) Physical principles of nuclear magnetic resonance. In: Newton TH, Potts DG (eds) Modern neuroradiology, vol 2. Advanced imaging techniques. Clavadel Press, San Anselmo, pp 15–61

Bradley WG (1987) Pathophysiologic correlates of signal alterations. In: Brant-Zawadski M, Norman D (eds) Magnetic resonance imaging of the central nervous system. Raven Press, New York, pp 23–42

Brant-Zawadski M (1987) Magnetic resonance imaging: the bare necessities. In: Brant-Zawadski M, Norman D (eds) Magnetic resonance imaging of the central nervous system. Raven Press, New York, pp 1–12

Bydder GM, Young IR (1985) Clinical use of the inversion recovery sequence. JCAT 9: 659

Crooks LE, Arakawa M, Hoenninger J et al. (1984) Magnetic resonance imaging: effects of magnetic field strength. Radiology 151: 127

Edelstein WA, Bottomley PA, Hart MR et al. (1983) Signal, noise and contrast in nuclear magnetic resonance (NMR) imaging. JCAT 7: 391

Edelstein WA, Glover GH, Hardy CJ et al. (1986) Intrinsic signal-to-noise ratio in NMR imaging. Magn Res Med 3: 604

Feinberg DA, Mills CM, Posin JP et al. (1985) Multiple spin echo magnetic resonance imaging. Radiology 155: 437

Fullerton GD, Cameron IL, Ord VA (1984) Frequency dependence of magnetic resonance spin-lattice relaxation of protons in biological materials. Radiology 151: 135

Heiken JP, Glazer HS, Lee JKT et al. (1987) Manual of clinical magnetic resonance imaging. A practical guide to conducting magnetic resonance imaging examinations of the head and body. Raven Press, New York

Hendrick RE, Nelson TR, Hendee WR (1984) Optimizing tissue contrast in magnetic resonance imaging. Magnetic Resonance Imaging 2: 193

Koenig SH, Brown RD, Adams D et al. (1984) Magnetic field dependence of 1/T1 of protons in tissue. Radiology 153: 858

Mitchell MR, Tarr RW, Conturo TE et al. (1986) Spin echo technique selection: basic principles for choosing MRI pulse sequence timing intervals. Radiographics 6: 245

Moran PR (1985) General approach to T1, T2 and spin-density discrimination sensitivities in NMR imaging sequences. Radiology 157: 284

Ortendahl DA, Hylton N, Kaufman L et al. (1984) Analytical tools for magnetic resonance imaging. Radiology 153: 479

Partain CL, Price RR, Rollo FD, James AE (eds) (1983) Nuclear magnetic resonance imaging. Saunders, Philadelphia

Partain CL, Price RR, Patton JA et al. (eds) (1987) Magnetic resonance imaging, 2nd edn. Saunders, Philadelphia (in press)

Perman WH, Hilal SK, Simon HE et al. (1985) Contrast manipulation in NMR imaging. Radiology 157: 285

Pykett IL, Newhouse JH, Buonanno FS et al. (1982) Principles of nuclear magnetic resonance imaging. Radiology 143: 157

Radiographics (1984) vol 4, Special Edition, Jan 1984

Shaw D (1987) Principles, methodology and applications of biomedical magnetic resonance. In: Wehrli FW, Shaw D, Kneeland B (eds), chapter 1. VCH Publishers, New York

Wehrli FW, McFall JR, Newton TH (1983) Parameters determining the appearance of NMR images. In: Newton TH, Potts DG (eds) Modern neuroradiology, vol 2. Advanced imaging techniques. Clavadel Press, San Anselmo, pp 81–117

Wehrli FW, McFall JR, Glover GH et al. (1984) Dependence of nuclear magnetic resonance (NMR) image contrast on intrinsic and pulse sequence timing parameters. Magnetic Resonance Imaging 2: 3

Wehrli FW, McFall JR, Shutts D et al. (1984) Mechanisms of contrast in NMR imaging. JCAT 8: 369

Young SW (1984) Nuclear magnetic resonance. Raven Press, New York

Clinical Results

See: Radiology (1987) RSNA index to imaging literature. Vol 162, part II.

Berquist TH (ed) (1987) Magnetic resonance of the musculoskeletal system. Raven Press, New York

Brant-Zawadski M, Norman D (eds) (1987) Magnetic resonance imaging of the central nervous system. Raven Press, New York

Stark DD, Bradley WG (eds) (1988) Magnetic resonance imaging. Mosby, Saint Louis

Technology

Bell RA (1987) Magnetic resonance instrumentation. In: Brant-Zawadski M, Norman D (eds) Magnetic resonance imaging of the central nervous system. Raven Press, New York, pp 13–22

King KF, Moran PR (1984) A unified description of NMR imaging data collection strategies and reconstruction. Med Phys 11: 1

Pickens DR, Erickson JJ (1985) Computers in computed tomography and magnetic resonance imaging. Radiographics 5: 31

Surface Coils

Ehman RL (1985) MR imaging with surface coils. Radiology 157: 549

Fischer MR, Barker B, Amparo BG et al. (1985) MR imaging using specialized coils. Radiology 157: 443

Roschmann P, Tischler R (1986) Surface coil proton MR imaging at 2T. Radiology 161: 251

Schenck JF, Foster TH, Henkes JL et al. (1985) High-field surface coil MR imaging of localized anatomy. AJNR 6: 181

Oblique Imaging

Edelman RR, Stark DD, Saini S et al. (1986) Oblique planes of section in MR imaging. Radiology 159: 809

Feiglin DH, George CR, MacIntyre WJ et al. (1985) Gated cardiac magnetic resonance structural imaging: optimization by electronic axial rotation. Radiology 154: 129

Hubert DJ, Mueller E, Heubes P (1985) Oblique magnetic resonance imaging of normal structures. AJR 145: 843

Fast Imaging

Frahm J, Haase A, Matthaei D (1986) Rapid NMR imaging using the FLASH technique. JCAT 10: 363

Haacke EM, Bearden FH, Clayton JR et al. (1986) Reduction of MR imaging time by the hybrid fast-scan technique. Radiology 158: 521

Mills TC, Ortendahl DA, Hylton NM et al. (1987) Partial flip angle MR imaging. Radiology 162: 531

Wehrli FW (1987) Introduction to fast-scan magnetic resonance. General Electric

Image Processing

Bobman SA, Riederer SJ, Lee JN et al. (1985) Synthetized MR images: comparison with acquired images. Radiology 155: 731

Bobman SA, Riederer SJ, Lee JN et al. (1986) Pulse sequence extrapolation with MR image synthesis. Radiology 159: 253

Crooks LE, Hylton NM, Ortendahl DA et al. (1987) The value of relaxation times and density measurements in clinical MRI. Invest Radiol (in press)

Kjos BO, Ehman RL, Brant-Zawadski M et al. (1985) Reproducibility of relaxation times and spin density calculated from MR imaging sequences: clinical study of the CNS. AJNR 6: 271

Majumdar S, Orphanoudakis SC, Gmitro A et al. (1986) Errors in the measurements of T2 using multiple-echo MRI techniques. Magn Res Med 3: 397, 562

Riederer SJ, Suddarth SA, Bobman SA et al. (1984) Automated MR image synthesis: feasibility studies. Radiology 153: 203

Blood Flow

Axel L (1984) Blood flow effects in magnetic resonance imaging. AJR 143: 1157

Bradley WG, Waluch V (1985) Blood flow: magnetic resonance imaging. Radiology 154: 443

Bradley WG (1987) Magnetic resonance appearance of flowing blood flow and cerebrospinal fluid. In: Brant-Zawadski M, Norman D (eds) Magnetic resonance imaging of the central nervous system. Raven Press, New York, pp 83–96

Dumoulin CL, Hart HR Jr (1986) Magnetic resonance angiography. Radiology 161: 717

Schulthess GK von, Higgins CB (1985) Magnetic resonance. Blood flow imaging with MR: spin-phase phenomena. Radiology 157: 687

Waluch V, Bradley WG (1984) NMR even echo rephasing in slow laminar flow. JCAT 8: 594

Paramagnetic Substances/Contrast Media

Drayer BP, Burger P, Darwin R et al. (1986) Magnetic resonance imaging of brain iron. AJNR 7: 373

Gomori JM, Grossman RI, Goldberg HI et al. (1985) Intracranial hematomas: imaging by high-field MR. Radiology 157: 87

Gomori JM, Grossman RI (1987) Head and neck hemorrhage. In: Kressel HY (ed) Magnetic resonance annual, 1987. Raven Press, New York, pp 71–117

Kabalka G, Buonocore E, Hubner K et al. (1987) Gadolinium-labeled liposomes: targeted agents for the liver and spleen. Radiology 163: 255

McNamara MT (1987) Paramagnetic contrast media for magnetic resonance imaging of the central nervous system. In: Brant-Zawadski M, Norman D (eds) Magnetic resonance imaging of the central nervous system. Raven Press, New York, pp 97–106

Norman D (1987) Vascular disease: hemorrhage. In: Brant-Zawadski M, Norman D (eds) Magnetic resonance imaging of the central nervous system. Raven Press, New York, pp 221–234

Saini S, Stark D, Hahn PF et al. (1987) Ferrite particles: a superparamagnetic MR contrast agent for the reticuloendothelial system. Radiology 162: 211

Weinmann HJ, Brasch RD, Press WR et al. (1984) Characteristics of gadolinium-DTPA complex: a potential NMR contrast agent. AJR 142: 619

Wolf GL, Burnett KR, Goldstein EJ et al. (1985) Contrast agents for magnetic resonance imaging. In: Kressel HY (ed) Magnetic resonance annual 1985. Raven Press, New York, pp 231–266

Cardiac and Respiratory Gating

Crooks LE, Barker B, Chang H et al. (1984) Magnetic resonance imaging strategies for heart studies. Radiology 153: 459

Ehman RL, McNamara MT, Pallack M et al. (1984) Magnetic resonance imaging with respiratory gating: techniques and advantages. AJR 143: 1175

Enzmann DR, Rubin JB et al. (1987) Use of cerebrospinal fluid gating to improve T2-weighted images. Radiology 162: 763

Lanzer P, Barta C, Botvinick EH et al. (1984) ECG-synchronized cardiac MR imaging: method and evaluation. Radiology 155: 681

Lanzer P, Botvinick EH, Schiller NB et al. (1984) Cardiac imaging using gated magnetic resonance. Radiology 150: 121

Lewis CE, Prato FS, Drost DJ et al. (1986) Comparison of respiratory triggering and gating techniques for the removal of respiratory artifacts in MR imaging. Radiology 160: 803

Runge RL, Clanton JA, Partain CL et al. (1984) Respiratory gating in magnetic resonance imaging at 0.5 Tesla. Radiology 151: 521

Artifacts

Babcock EE, Libby B, Weinreb JC et al. (1985) Edge artifacts in MR images: chemical shift effect. JCAT 9: 252

Bellon EM, Haacke EM, Coleman PE et al. (1986) MR artifacts: a review. AJR 147: 1271

Dwyer AJ, Knop RH, Hoult DI (1985) Frequency shift artifacts in MR imaging. JCAT 9: 16

Kelly WM (1987) Image artifacts and technical limitations. In: Brant-Zawadski M, Norman D (eds) Magnetic resonance imaging of the central nervous system. Raven Press, New York, pp 43–82

Lufkin RB, Pusey E, Stark DD et al. (1986) Boundary artifacts due to truncation errors in MR imaging. AJR 147: 1283

Pele NJ, Glover GH, Charles HC (1985) Respiration artifacts in MRI. In: Proceedings of the Society of Magnetic Resonance in Medicine, Aug 19–23, London

Perman WH, Moran PR, Moran RA et al. (1986) Artifacts from pulsatile flow in MR imaging. JCAT 10: 473

Pusey E, Lufkin RB, Brown RKJ et al. (1986) Magnetic resonance imaging artifacts: mechanisms and clinical significance. Radiographics 6: 891

Schultz CL, Alfidi RJ, Nelson AD et al. (1984) The effect of motion on two-dimensional Fourier transformation magnetic resonance images. Radiology 152: 117

Biological Effects/Safety

Bottomley PA, Andrew ER (1978) RF magnetic field penetration, phase shift and power dissipation in biological tissue: implication for NMR imaging. Phys Med Biol 23: 630

Davis PL, Crooks LE, Arakawa M et al. (1981) Potential hazards in NMR imaging: heating effects of changing magnetic fields on small metallic implants. AJR 137: 857

National Radiological Protection Board Ad Hoc Advisory Group on Nuclear Magnetic Resonance Imaging (1983) Revised guidance on acceptable limits of exposure during nuclear magnetic resonance clinical imaging. Br J Radiol 56: 974

New PFJ, Rosen BR, Brady TJ et al. (1983) Potential hazards and artifacts of ferromagnetic and nonferromagnetic surgical and dental materials and devices in nuclear magnetic resonance imaging. Radiology 147: 139

Pavlicek W, Geisinger M, Castle L et al. (1985) The effects of nuclear magnetic resonance in patients with cardiac pacemakers. Radiology 147: 149

Shellock FG, Schaefer DF, Gordon CJ (1986) Effect of a 1.5 T static magnetic field on body temperature on man. Magn Reson Med 3: 644

Shellock FG, Crues JV (1987) Temperature, heart rate, and blood pressure changes associated with clinical MR imaging at 1.5 T. Radiology 163: 259

Soulen RL, Budinger TF, Higgins CB (1985) Magnetic resonance imaging of prosthetic heart valves. Radiology 154: 705

Patient Preparation

Finn EJ, Di Chiro G, Brooks RA et al. (1985) Ferromagnetic materials in patients: detection before MR imaging. Radiology 156: 139

Hricak H, Amparo EG (1984) Body MRI: alleviation of claustrophobia by prone position. Radiology 152: 819

Weinreb JC, Maravilla KR, Peshock R et al. (1984) Magnetic resonance imaging: improving patient tolerance and safety. AJR 143: 1285

Subject Index

Acquisition time 64
Air 6, 50
Aliasing 92
Artifacts 89-92

Bo: see magnetic field
Bone 50

Calcifications 50
Chemical shift 92
Coil 8, 59
Console 57
Contraindications 55
Contrast media 86

Echo
- formation 25
- gradient reversal echo 33, 94
- multiple spin echo 27
- spin echo 23
- symmetrical/asymmetrical echo 29
Electromagnetic wave 2
Encoding 94
Energy 2
- level 9
Equilibrium 8
Excitation 8

Facility (MR) 56
Faraday (cage) 57
Fast imaging 33
Field of view 60
Flow effects 78

Gadolinium 86
Gating 89
Gauss 9
Gradient
- coil 93
- magnetic field 93
Grey scale 61
Gyromagnetic ratio 93

Image (MR)
- quality 62
- synthetic 50
Imaging plane 37, 93
IR (inversion recovery) 30

Larmor (frequency) 93

Magnet 9
Magnetic field 8, 62
- gradients 93
- inhomogeneities 14
Magnetization vector M 9
Matrix 61
Multislice imaging 65

Noise: see signal/noise ratio
Nucleus 1

Paramagnetic substances 86
Partial saturation 22
Phase 12, 14
Pixel 61
Precession 13
- cone 13
Proton 1
Proton density (ρ) 6, 22, 26, 29, 30
Pulse
- radiofrequency 19
- sequence 20

Radiofrequency 2
Relaxation times 6-15
- quantitative analysis 50
- spin lattice or longitudinal: see T1
- spin spin or transversal: see T2
Resonance 9

Safety 55
Sequences (MR) 21-35
- choice 43
- fast imaging 33
- inversion recovery 30
- partial saturation 22